Julia B. Hennermann

Neue Erkenntnisse und Strategien in der Behandlung der Phenylketonurie

Julia B. Hennermann

Neue Erkenntnisse und Strategien in der Behandlung der Phenylketonurie

Südwestdeutscher Verlag für Hochschulschriften

Impressum / Imprint
Bibliografische Information der Deutschen Nationalbibliothek: Die Deutsche Nationalbibliothek verzeichnet diese Publikation in der Deutschen Nationalbibliografie; detaillierte bibliografische Daten sind im Internet über http://dnb.d-nb.de abrufbar.
Alle in diesem Buch genannten Marken und Produktnamen unterliegen warenzeichen-, marken- oder patentrechtlichem Schutz bzw. sind Warenzeichen oder eingetragene Warenzeichen der jeweiligen Inhaber. Die Wiedergabe von Marken, Produktnamen, Gebrauchsnamen, Handelsnamen, Warenbezeichnungen u.s.w. in diesem Werk berechtigt auch ohne besondere Kennzeichnung nicht zu der Annahme, dass solche Namen im Sinne der Warenzeichen- und Markenschutzgesetzgebung als frei zu betrachten wären und daher von jedermann benutzt werden dürften.

Bibliographic information published by the Deutsche Nationalbibliothek: The Deutsche Nationalbibliothek lists this publication in the Deutsche Nationalbibliografie; detailed bibliographic data are available in the Internet at http://dnb.d-nb.de.
Any brand names and product names mentioned in this book are subject to trademark, brand or patent protection and are trademarks or registered trademarks of their respective holders. The use of brand names, product names, common names, trade names, product descriptions etc. even without a particular marking in this works is in no way to be construed to mean that such names may be regarded as unrestricted in respect of trademark and brand protection legislation and could thus be used by anyone.

Coverbild / Cover image: www.ingimage.com

Verlag / Publisher:
Südwestdeutscher Verlag für Hochschulschriften
ist ein Imprint der / is a trademark of
OmniScriptum GmbH & Co. KG
Heinrich-Böcking-Str. 6-8, 66121 Saarbrücken, Deutschland / Germany
Email: info@svh-verlag.de

Herstellung: siehe letzte Seite /
Printed at: see last page
ISBN: 978-3-8381-3779-7

Zugl. / Approved by: Berlin, Charité Universitätsmedizin Berlin, Habilitationsschrift, 2013

Copyright © 2014 OmniScriptum GmbH & Co. KG
Alle Rechte vorbehalten. / All rights reserved. Saarbrücken 2014

Inhaltsverzeichnis

Häufig benutzte Abkürzungen 3
1. Einleitung 4
1.1. Enzymdefekt bei Phenylketonurie 4
1.2. Klinische Symptome unbehandelter Patienten mit Phenylketonurie 5
1.3. Diagnosestellung der Phenylketonurie 5
1.4. Klassifizierung der Phenylketonurie 6
1.5. Prävalenz und Vererbung der Phenylketonurie 7
1.6. Behandlung der Phenylketonurie 7
2. Eigene Arbeiten 10
2.1. PUBLIKATION 1: Hennermann JB, Vetter B, Wolf C, Windt E, Bührdel P, Seidl J, Mönch E, Kulozik AE. Phenylketonuria and Hyperphenylalaninemia in Eastern Germany: A Characteristic Molecular Profile and 15 Novel Mutations. 2000. Hum Mutat 15:254-260. DOI 10.1002/(SICI)1098-1004(200003)15:3<254::AID-HUMU6>3.0.CO;2-W 10
2.2. PUBLIKATION 2: Hennermann JB, Roloff S, Gellermann J, Vollmer I, Windt E, Vetter B, Plöckinger U, Mönch E, Querfeld U. Chronic Kidney Disease in Adolescent and Adult Patients with Phenylketonuria. 2013. J Inherit Metab Dis 36:747–756. DOI 10.1007/s10545-012-9548-0 19
2.3. PUBLIKATION 3: Hennermann JB, Bührer C, Blau N, Vetter B, Mönch E. Long-term treatment with tetrahydrobiopterin increases phenylalanine tolerance in children with severe phenotype of phenylketonuria. 2005. Mol Genet Metab 86:S86-S90. DOI 10.1016/j.ymgme.2005.05.013 32
2.4. PUBLIKATION 4: Trefz FK, Burton BK, Longo N, Martinez-Pardo Casanova M, Gruskin DJ, Dorenbaum A, Kakkis ED, Crombez EA, Grange DK, Harmatz P, Levy HL, Lipson MH, Milanowski A, Randolph LM, Vockley G, Whitley CB, Wolff JA, Bebchuk J, Christ-Schmidt H, Hennermann JB. Efficacy of sapropterin dihydrochloride in increasing phenylalanine tolerance in children with phenylketonuria: a Phase III, randomized, double-blind, placebo-controlled study. 2009. J Pediatr 154:700-707. DOI 10.1016/j.jpeds.2008.11.040 38
2.5. PUBLIKATION 5: Burton BK, Nowacka M, Hennermann JB, Lipson M, Grange DK, Chakrapani A, Trefz F, Dorenbaum A, Imperiale M, Kim SS, Fernhoff PM. Safety of Extended Treatment with Sapropterin Dihydrochloride in Patients with Phenylketonuria: Results of a Phase 3b Study. 2011. Mol Genet Metab 103:315-322. DOI 10.1016/j.ymgme.2011.03.020 49
2.6. PUBLIKATION 6: Hennermann JB, Roloff S, Gebauer C, Vetter B, von Arnim-Baas A, Mönch E. Long-term treatment with tetrahydrobiopterin in phenylketonuria: Treatment strategies and prediction of long-term responders. 2012. Mol Genet Metab 107:294-301. DOI 10.1016/j.ymgme.2012.09.021 58

2.7. PUBLIKATION 7: Blau N, Hennermann JB, Langenbeck U, Lichter-Konecki U. Diagnosis, Classification, and Genetics of Phenylketonuria and Tetrahydrobiopterin (BH4) Deficiencies. 2011. Mol Genet Metab 104:S2-S9. DOI 10.1016/j.ymgme.2011.08.017 68

3. Diskussion 77

3.1. Phenylalanin-bilanzierte diätetische Therapie 77

3.1.1. Langzeitprobleme unter Phenylalanin-bilanzierter Diät 77

3.1.2. Nierenfunktion bei Patienten mit Phenylalanin-bilanzierter Diät 78

3.1.3. Genese der Nierenschädigung unter Phenylalanin-bilanzierter Diät 79

3.2. Therapie mit Tetrahydrobiopterin (BH4) 81

3.2.1. Identifikation von langzeit-BH4-responsiven PKU-Patienten 82

3.2.2. Prädiktive Parameter für Langzeit-BH4-Responsivität 84

3.2.3. Langzeittherapie mit Tetrahydrobiopterin (BH4) 85

3.3. Ausblick 87

4. Zusammenfassung 88

5. Literaturangaben aus dem freien Text 90

Danksagung 98

Häufig benutzte Abkürzungen

BH4	6R-5,6,7,8-Tetrahydrobiopterin
GFR	Glomeruläre Filtrationsrate
GMP	Glykomakropeptide
HPA	Hyperphenylalaninämie
KG	Körpergewicht
LNAA	Lange neutrale Aminosäuren
PAH	Phenylalanin-4-Hydroxylase
Phe	Phenylalanin
PKU	Phenylketonurie
Sapropterin	Sapropterin-Dihydrochlorid
Tyr	Tyrosin

1. Einleitung

Die Phenylketonurie (PKU, MIM 261600) ist die häufigste angeborene Störung im Aminosäurenstoffwechsel und die erste angeborene Stoffwechselerkrankung, bei der eine diätetische Therapie etabliert wurde (Scriver und Kaufman 2001). Obwohl die diätetische Therapie bereits in den 1950er Jahren erstmals beschrieben wurde (Bickel et al. 1953), hat sich in der Behandlung der PKU jahrzehntelang wenig verändert. Erst in den letzten Jahren begann die erfolgreiche Suche nach neuen Therapieoptionen zur Behandlung der PKU.

1.1. Enzymdefekt bei Phenylketonurie

Ursächlich für die PKU ist eine Defizienz der Phenylalanin-4-Hydroxylase (PAH, EC 1.14.16.1) (Scriver und Kaufman 2001). Die PAH katalysiert die Hydroxilierung von Phenylalanin (Phe) zu Tyrosin (Tyr) unter Mithilfe des aktiven Pterins 6R-5,6,7,8-Tetrahydrobiopterin (BH4) als Kofaktor, molekularem Sauerstoff und Eisen (s. Abbildung 1). BH4 wird in drei Schritten aus Guanosintriphosphat synthetisiert, über eine Hydroxilierungsreaktion in das inaktive Pterin-4α-Carbinolamin umgewandelt und dann mittels zweier Enzyme über Dihydrobiopterin regeneriert (Walter et al. 2006). Sowohl eine PAH-Defizienz als auch Defekte in der Synthese oder Regeneration von BH4 resultieren in einem Anstieg der Phe-Blutkonzentrationen. Normale Phe-Blutkonzentrationen liegen im Neugeborenenalter bei ≤180 µmol/L, ab dem 3. Lebensmonat bei ≤130 µmol/L (Clayton et al. 1980).

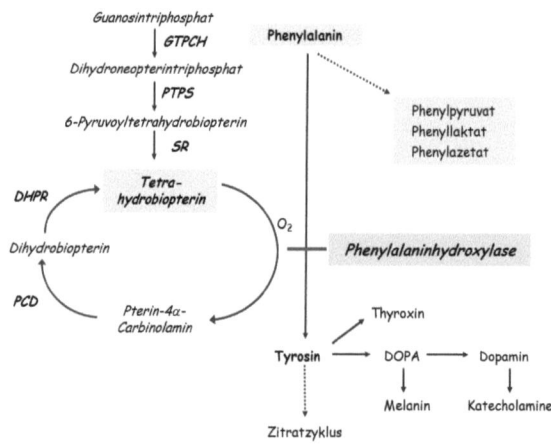

Abbildung 1: Abbaustörung bei Phenylketonurie *(nach Mönch et al. 2006, Walter et al. 2002)*

1.2. Klinische Symptome unbehandelter Patienten mit Phenylketonurie

Kinder mit PKU sind bei Geburt klinisch unauffällig. Unbehandelt führt die Erkrankung jedoch zu einer irreversiblen schweren Hirnschädigung, resultierend in geistiger Behinderung (IQ zwischen 30-50), Mikrozephalie, EEG-Veränderungen, zerebralen Krampfanfällen, Pyramidenbahnzeichen, Tremor und Verhaltensstörungen. Durch den Mangel an Tyrosin und die verminderte Bildung von Melanin weisen nicht-behandelte PKU-Patienten eine Pigmentarmut der Haut und Haare auf. Typisch ist zudem ein den Patienten eigener „mäuseartiger" Geruch, bedingt durch den Anstau von Phenylketonen (Pitt 1971, Scriver und Kaufman 2001).

Die Aufklärung des Pathomechanismus der Hirnschädigung bei Patienten mit PKU ist Gegenstand vieler Studien. Eine wichtige Rolle spielt der L-Aminosäuren-Transporter LAT1 an der Bluthirnschranke. Der LAT1-Transporter bindet selektiv an lange neutrale Aminosäuren (LNAA) (Boado et al. 1999, Choi und Pardridge 1986). Zu den LNAA zählen Tryptophan, die verzweigtkettigen Aminosäuren Valin, Isoleucin und Leucin sowie Tyrosin und Phenylalanin (Matalon et al. 2007). Da die Bindung der LNAA an den LAT1-Transporter einem kompetitiven Prozess folgt, führen hohe Phe-Blutkonzentrationen zu einer verminderten Aufnahme anderer LNAA über die Bluthirnschranke (Pietz et al. 1999). Intrazerebral resultieren daher bei PKU-Patienten mit hohen Phe-Blutkonzentrationen erniedrigte Konzentrationen anderer LNAA, insbesondere der von Tyrosin und Tryptophan (McKean 1972, Pietz et al. 1999). Dies bedingt eine verminderte Synthese der Neurotransmitter Dopamin, Noradrenalin und Serotonin (Burlina et al. 2000, Butler et al. 1981, McKean 1972), aber auch eine Hemmung der zerebralen Proteinsynthese mit folgender Myelinisierungsstörung (Bauman und Kemper 1982, Binek-Singer und Johnson 1982, Hughes und Johnson 1978). Beides scheint hauptsächlich für die kognitiven Störungen bei Patienten mit PKU zu sein (de Groot et al. 2010). In den letzten Jahren konnten zudem weitere Faktoren identifiziert werden, die einen Einfluss auf die Hirnschädigung bei Patienten mit unbehandelter PKU haben: Hohe intrazerebrale Phe-Konzentrationen interagieren mit dem neuronalen Zelladhäsionsmolekül L1 CAM sowie mit Peroxisom-Proliferator-aktivierten Rezeptoren (PPARγ). Dies scheint zu einem verminderten Neuritenwachstum und zur Apoptose zu führen (Hartwig et al. 2006, Schumacher et al. 2008).

1.3. Diagnosestellung der Phenylketonurie

Die PKU wurde erstmals 1934 von dem Norweger Ivar Asbjørn Følling beschrieben (Følling 1934). Følling erkannte den Zusammenhang zwischen der Ausscheidung von Phenylpyruvat im Urin und einer mentalen Retardierung. Der Nachweis von Phenylpyruvat gelang Følling mittels des Eisen(III)-Chlorid-Tests. Dieser sogenannte „Windeltest" wird bei Phe-Blutwerten >900 µmol/L positiv und war die erste Methode zur Diagnose einer PKU (Böhles et al. 1999).

1963 wurde von dem amerikanischen Mikrobiologen Robert Guthrie erstmals das Screening auf Phenylketonurie aus getrockneten Blutstropfen mit Hilfe des Bakterien-Hemmtests beschrieben (Guthrie und Susi 1963). Diese Methode wurde als Neugeborenenscreening kurze Zeit später auch in Deutschland etabliert: in der BRD im Jahr 1969 und in der DDR im Jahr 1971 (Mathias und Bickel 1986, Machill et al. 1994). Seit 2005 wird die PKU bundesweit durch das standardisierte erweiterte Neugeborenenscreening mittels Tandem-Massenspektrometrie erfasst (BAnz 2005). Durch eine frühe Diagnosestellung im Neugeborenenscreening und einen rechtzeitigen Therapiebeginn wird bei Patienten mit PKU eine mentale Retardierung verhindert und eine weitgehend normale Entwicklung gewährleistet. Das langfristige Outcome ist jedoch im Wesentlichen abhängig von der individuellen Stoffwechseleinstellung (Waisbren et al. 2007).

1.4. Klassifizierung der Phenylketonurie

Abhängig von dem Genotyp, von der PAH-Restenzymaktivität und somit von der Schwere der Erkrankung sind verschiedene Verlaufsformen der PKU mit unterschiedlichen Phänotypen beschrieben. In den deutschsprachigen Ländern erfolgt die Klassifizierung der PKU in drei unterschiedliche Phänotypen: die klassische PKU, die milde PKU und die Hyperphenylalaninämie (HPA). Sowohl die klassische wie auch die milde PKU sind behandlungspflichtig, während Individuen mit einer HPA keine Therapie benötigen, da ihre Phe-Blutwerte auch unter normaler Kost nicht >600 µmol/L ansteigen und keine Gefahr einer neurologischen Schädigung besteht (Weglage et al. 1996). Die Einteilung in die verschiedenen PKU-Phänotypen erfolgt nach etablierten Kriterien anhand der maximalen Phe-Blutwerte vor Therapiebeginn und der täglichen Phe-Toleranz (Guldberg et al. 1998, Güttler et al. 1994) (Tabelle 1).

Tabelle 1: Einteilung der verschiedenen PKU-Phänotypen nach klinischen Kriterien

PKU-Phänotyp	Maximaler Phe-Wert im Blut	Phe-Toleranz
Klassische PKU	>1.200 µmol/L	<20 mg/kg/die
Milde PKU	600 - 1.200 µmol/L	20 - 50 mg/kg/die
HPA	<600 µmol/L	>50 mg/kg/die

1.5. Prävalenz und Vererbung der Phenylketonurie

Die Häufigkeit der PKU weist unterschiedliche geographische Verteilungen auf, auch innerhalb Europas. Nach den aktuellen Daten der Deutschen Gesellschaft für Neugeborenenscreening liegt die Prävalenz aller PKU-Formen in Deutschland bei 1: 5.000. Im Jahr 2010 wurden im Neugeborenenscreening in der Bundesrepublik Deutschland folgende Prävalenzen erfasst: klassische und milde PKU 1: 9.287; HPA 1: 11.114; BH4-Mangel 1: 677.947; Gesamtzahl 1: 5.022 (*http://www.screening-dgns.de*).

Die Vererbung der PKU folgt einem autosomal-rezessiven Erbgang. Das *PAH*-Gen ist auf 12q21-q24.1 lokalisiert, besteht aus 13 Exonen und kodiert 452 Aminosäuren (DiLella et al. 1986, Scriver und Kaufman 2001). Derzeit sind über 700 verschiedene *PAH*-Mutationen beschrieben. Davon sind 61% Missense-Mutationen, 14% Deletionen, 11% Spleißstellen-Mutationen, 6% stille Mutationen, 5% Nonsense-Mutationen und 2% Insertionen. Alle diese bekannten *PAH*-Mutationen sind in einer Gen-Datenbank zusammengefasst (*http://www.pahdb.mcgill.ca*). PAH liegt in seiner funktionellen Form als Homotetramer vor. Das tetramere Enzym weist drei unterschiedliche Domänen auf: eine regulatorische Domäne, eine katalytische Domäne sowie eine tetramerisierende Domäne. Das aktive Zentrum der PAH liegt in der katalytischen Domäne (Erlandsen und Stevens 1999). Je nachdem, welchen Einfluss die *PAH*-Mutationen auf die Struktur des Tetramers haben, sind diese mit unterschiedlichen Rest-Enzymaktivitäten und daraus folgend mit unterschiedlichen klinischen Phänotypen assoziiert (Erlandsen und Stevens 1999).

1.6. Behandlung der Phenylketonurie

Zur Verhinderung neurologischer Schädigungen ist bei Patienten mit PKU eine lebenslange Therapie indiziert (MacDonald et al. 2010). Abhängig von dem Lebensalter sind international unterschiedliche Therapieziele zur Behandlung der PKU etabliert. Die in Deutschland aktuell gültigen altersabhängigen Phe-Zielwerte im Blut sind der Tabelle 2 zu entnehmen (Burgard et al.1999).

Tabelle 2: Phe-Zielwerte nach den aktuellen Empfehlungen zur Behandlung der PKU

Alter	Phe-Zielwerte im Blut
<10 Jahre	40 - 240 µmol/L
10 - 15 Jahre	40 - 900 µmol/L
>15 Jahre	40 - 1.200 µmol/L

Diätetische Behandlung

1953 wurde von dem Deutschen Horst Bickel erstmals die Behandlung der PKU beschrieben. Die Behandlung des zweijährigen Mädchens Sheila mit einem Phe-freien Aminosäurenhydrolysat wurde von Bickel in seiner Arbeit „*Influence of phenylalanine intake on phenylketonuria*" dargestellt (Bickel et al. 1953). Auch heute noch stellt die Diät die Basis der PKU-Behandlung dar. Grundlage ist eine streng Phe-bilanzierte Diät mit Substitution eines synthetischen Phe-freien L-Aminosäurengemisches (MacDonald et al. 2011, Scriver und Kaufmann 2001). Die diätetische Behandlung der PKU wurde in den letzten Jahrzehnten kontinuierlich verbessert, insbesondere durch eine Optimierung des Geschmacks und der Zusammensetzung der Aminosäuregemische sowie durch ein stark erweitertes Angebot eiweißarmer Nahrungsmittel. Dennoch ist die Diäteinhaltung für viele Patienten eine große Herausforderung, und die Compliance nimmt häufig im Laufe der Behandlung ab, insbesondere im Adoleszenten- und Erwachsenenalter (MacDonald et al. 2010, Walter et al. 2002).

Alternative Behandlungsoptionen

Erst in den letzten Jahren begann die erfolgreiche Suche nach neuen Therapieoptionen zur Behandlung der PKU. Eine dieser Therapieoptionen ist die Behandlung mit LNAA. Das Prinzip der Behandlung besteht darin, dass LNAA den gleichen LAT1-Transporter wie Phe benutzen, und zwar sowohl an der Bluthirnschranke als auch im Gastrointestinaltrakt (Boado et al. 1999, Choi und Pardridge 1986, Hidalgo und Borchardt 1990). Die Gabe von LNAA senkt daher einerseits die Phe-Konzentration im Blut durch eine verminderte Phe-Aufnahme im Gastrointestinaltrakt und hat andererseits einen neuroprotektiven Effekt durch eine verminderte Phe- und eine erhöhte LNAA-Aufnahme über die Bluthirnschranke. Die Therapie mit LNAA findet ausschließlich Anwendung bei erwachsenen Patienten und ist keine Therapieoption für Kinder und Jugendliche mit PKU (Ahring 2010, Matalon et al. 2007, Schindeler et al. 2007). LNAA-Präparate sind in Deutschland derzeit nicht verfügbar.

Eine andere neue Therapieoption ist die Behandlung mit Glykomakropeptiden (GMP). GMP sind Teile des Molkeproteins und enthalten als einziges natürliches Protein nur sehr geringe Mengen an Phe (2,5-5 mg Phe/g Protein). Zudem haben GMP einen hohen Gehalt an LNAA, der zwei- bis dreifach höher ist als in anderem natürlichen Protein (van Calcar et al. 2009). Als hochwertiges und schmackhaftes Protein stellen GMP eine gute Proteinquelle für die PKU-Behandlung dar, jedoch nur bei Substitution der in GMP fehlenden essentiellen Aminosäuren. Bislang wurden GMP vorwiegend in Studien angewandt, hierbei zeigte sich unter der Gabe von GMP insbesondere ein verbesserter Phe-Umsatz, eine Erleichterung der Diät sowie eine Verbesserung der Compliance (Lim et al. 2007, van Calcar et al. 2009).

Ein weiterer Therapieansatz ist die Enzymersatztherapie mit Phenylalanin-Ammonium-Lyase. Die Phenylalanin-Ammonium-Lyase ist kein humanes sondern ein pflanzliches Enzym, das die Umwandlung von Phe zu dem nicht-toxischen Metaboliten *trans*-Zimtsäure katalysiert (Gamez et al. 2005). Da eine Enzymersatztherapie mit Phenylalanin-Ammonium-Lyase ein hohes Risiko allergischer Reaktionen birgt, ist für die Therapie eine Konjugation der Phenylalanin-Ammonium-Lyase mit Polyethylenglycol („PEGylation") erforderlich (Gamez et al. 2005, Sarkissian et al. 2008). Derzeit werden erste klinische Studien mit der Enzymersatztherapie mit PEGylierter Phenylalanin-Ammonium-Lyase bei erwachsenen Patienten mit PKU durchgeführt (*http://clinicaltrials.gov*).

Die zellbasierte Therapie stellt eine weitere Alternative in der Behandlung der PKU dar. Kürzlich wurde bei einem ersten Patienten mit PKU bei ausgeprägter Incompliance und schlechter Stoffwechseleinstellung eine Hepatozytentransplantation durchgeführt, die jedoch nur zu einem kurzzeitigen Therapieerfolg führte (Stéphenne et al. 2012). Diese Therapiealternative scheint aufgrund der Invasivität sowie der potentiellen Nebenwirkungen keine wirkliche Alternative in der Behandlung der PKU darzustellen. Weitere Therapieoptionen werden derzeit am PKU-Mausmodell erprobt. Die Gentherapie mit Adeno-asoziierten Virus-Vektoren, die entweder in der Leber oder im Muskel exprimiert werden, zeigen im PKU-Mausmodell erfolgversprechende Ergebnisse mit langfristiger Korrektur der klinischen wie auch der laborchemischen Auffälligkeiten (Thöny 2010).

Behandlung mit Tetrahydrobiopterin (BH4)

Eine weitere Therapieoption ist die Gabe von BH4, dem Kofaktor der PAH, die erstmals von Kure und Mitarbeitern im Jahr 1999 beschrieben wurde (Kure et al. 1999). Sie berichteten über vier Patienten mit einer Erhöhung der Phe-Blutkonzentrationen, die keinen Defekt der BH4-Synthese oder -Regeneration sondern eine Defizienz der PAH aufwiesen und dennoch nach der Gabe von BH4 einen deutlichen Abfall ihrer Phe-Werte zeigten. Alle vier Patienten waren compound-heterozygot für Mutationen im *PAH*-Gen. Diese PKU-Form wird *BH4-responsive PKU* genannt. In der letzten Dekade wurden zahlreiche Patienten mit einer BH4-responsiven PKU beschrieben (Bernegger und Blau 2002, Levy et al. 2007, Muntau et al. 2002, Trefz et al. 2010). Die Mehrzahl dieser Patienten wies einen milden PKU-Phänotyp auf. Die Therapie mit BH4 stellt neben der lebenseinschränkenden Phe-bilanzierten Diät die erste zugelassene alternative Behandlungsoption für Kinder und Jugendliche mit einer PKU dar.

Im Folgenden werden in dieser Arbeit Langzeitprobleme bei der diätetischen Behandlung der PKU sowie Besonderheiten der Langzeittherapie mit BH4 evaluiert.

2. Eigene Arbeiten

2.1. PUBLIKATION 1: **Hennermann JB**, Vetter B, Wolf C, Windt E, Bührdel P, Seidel J, Mönch E, Kulozik AE. Phenylketonuria and Hyperphenylalaninemia in Eastern Germany: A Characteristic Molecular Profile and 15 Novel Mutations. 2000. Hum Mutat 15:254-260. DOI 10.1002/(SICI)1098-1004(200003)15:3<254::AID-HUMU6> 3.0.CO;2-W

Reprinted from: Human Mutation 2000, Volume 15 (3), page 254-60, with permission from John Wiley and Sons Inc., 2000, provided by Copyright Clearance Center

Ziel dieser Studie war die Untersuchung der Besonderheiten des genotypischen Spektrums der PKU-Patienten aus dem Ostteil Deutschlands. Wir untersuchten 302 Patienten aus 290 Familien, die in den Stoffwechselzentren Berlin, Leipzig und Jena betreut wurden. Insgesamt identifizierten wir 75 verschiedene Mutationen, von denen 15 Mutationen bislang nicht beschrieben waren. Von diesen 15 neu identifizierten Mutationen waren elf Punktmutationen (p.M1R, p.Q20L, p.L41P, p.R155P, p.E183Q, p.S231F, p.Y325C, p.E330D, p.G344R, p.G344V, p.F410S), eine Spleiß-Mutation (IVS9+1G>A) und drei Deletionen (c.737delC, c.838del8bp, c.1357-1361del). Elf dieser neu identifizierten Mutationen waren mit einer klassischen PKU, drei mit einer milden PKU und nur eine Mutation mit einer HPA assoziiert.

Bei der phänotypischen Klassifizierung zeigte sich ein sehr hoher Anteil an Patienten mit einer klassischen PKU (77% aller untersuchten Patienten); lediglich 14% der Patienten wiesen eine milde PKU und 9% eine HPA auf. Bei der Untersuchung des *PAH*-Genotyps bestätigte sich demnach eine hohe Frequenz an Nullmutationen. Zudem zeigten sich deutliche Unterschiede zwischen der PKU-Population ohne und der PKU-Population mit Migrationshintergrund. Bei der ostdeutschen PKU-Population ohne Migrationshintergrund war die Nullmutation p.R408W in 40% aller Allele nachweisbar, die Spleiß-Mutationen IVS12+1G>A und IVS10-11G>A in 8% bzw. 3% nachweisbar. Bei PKU-Patienten mit türkischem Migrationshintergrund wurden am häufigsten die beiden Spleiß-Mutationen IVS10-11G>A (57% aller Allele) und IVS2+5G>C (15% aller Allele) identifiziert. Keiner der PKU-Patienten mit türkischem Migrationshintergrund wies die in der deutschen Population häufigen Mutationen p.R408W oder IVS12+1G>A auf. Unterschiedliche Häufigkeiten der *PAH*-Mutationen sind bereits innerhalb Europas beschrieben (Eisensmith et al. 1995, Zschocke et al. 1997) und konnten anhand unserer Daten auch für Deutschland bestätigt werden.

Auffallend waren in der hier untersuchten PKU-Population die hohe Inzidenz an Patienten mit einer klassischen PKU und der sehr hohe Anteil an Nullmutationen im *PAH*-Gen. Die Bestimmung des Genotyps und somit auch die Prädiktion des daraus resultierenden Phänotyps sind essentiell für Entscheidungen über mögliche Therapieoptionen, wie im Folgenden dargestellt wird.

RESEARCH ARTICLE

Phenylketonuria and Hyperphenylalaninemia in Eastern Germany: A Characteristic Molecular Profile and 15 Novel Mutations

Julia B. Hennermann,[1] Barbara Vetter,[1] Claudia Wolf,[2] Elke Windt,[1] Peter Bührdel,[3] Jörg Seidel,[4] Eberhard Mönch,[1] and Andreas E. Kulozik[1]*

[1]*Children's Hospital, Charité Medical Center, Humboldt University, Berlin, Germany*
[2]*Department of Human Genetics, University of Leipzig, Leipzig, Germany*
[3]*Children's Hospital, University of Leipzig, Leipzig, Germany*
[4]*Children's Hospital, University of Jena, Jena, Germany*

Communicated by Mark Paalman

Phenylketonuria (PKU) is an important error of amino acid metabolism which results in most patients from phenylalanine hydroxylase (PAH) deficiency. PKU displays a marked genotypic heterogeneity both within and between different populations. The aim of this study was to establish the genotypic spectrum of PKU in eastern Germany, and to compare this to the distribution of mutations in western Germany. The study population included 302 patients in 290 families who were followed at treatment centers in Berlin, Leipzig and Jena. The study showed marked genotypic variability with a total of 75 mutations, including 15 that have so far not been described (eleven missense mutations, one splicing mutation, and three small deletions). One of these novel mutations, E183Q, occurred in cis to a R408W mutation. In the non-immigrant eastern German population, the frequency of R408W accounted for 40.1% of the PKU alleles. In the immigrant Turkish population of the former West Berlin, the most prevalent mutation was IVS10-11G>A (57%). There was a marked difference of the genotypic spectrum between the population studied here and the data reported from the western part of the country. Hum Mutat 15:254–260, 2000. © 2000 Wiley-Liss, Inc.

KEY WORDS: hyperphenylalaninemia; phenylketonuria; PAH; phenylalanine hydroxylase; eastern Germany

INTRODUCTION

Deficiency of hepatic phenylalanine hydroxylase (PAH; MIM# 251580) is the most common inborn error of amino acid metabolism. The clinical expression varies from a severe phenotype, phenylketonuria (PKU; MIM# 261600), to a mild form not requiring treatment, hyperphenylalaninemia (HPA). The identification of PAH gene mutations and the estimation of the corresponding residual enzyme activity is important to understand the allelic heterogeneity and the clinical variability of the phenotypes [Okano et al., 1991].

There are more than 300 known PAH gene mutations [Nowacki et al., 1998; Scriver et al., 2000], only a limited number of which are common in different populations. The genetic diversity of PKU in Europe is dominated by three mutations: the missense mutation R408W, which predominates in eastern Europe [Baranovskaya et al., 1996; Kozak et al., 1997; Schuler et al., 1994; Zygulska et al., 1991] and Great Britain [Eisensmith et al., 1995; Zschocke et al., 1997]; the splice mutation IVS12+1G>A in northern Europe [Guldberg et al., 1993; Svensson et al., 1993]; and the splice mutation IVS10-11G>A in southern Europe [Desviat et al., 1997; Guzzetta et al., 1997; Pérez et al., 1997; Özalp et al., 1994]. The data for Germany, most of which originated from the western part of the country before reunification, show that the two mutations IVS12+1G>A (25%; 11%) and R408W (20%; 19%), are the most common [Okano et al., 1991; Guldberg et al., 1996].

Received 9 September 1999; accepted revised manuscript 5 November 1999.

Correspondence to: Andreas E. Kulozik, Children's Hospital, Charité Medical Center, Augustenburger Platz 1, D-13353 Berlin, Germany. E-mail: andreas.kulozik@charite.de

© 000 WILEY-LISS, INC.

The molecular and basic clinical data in this report are presented from 290 PKU families who live in the eastern part of Germany and who are followed by the treatment centers in Berlin, Leipzig and Jena. Surprisingly, the spectrum of mutations is significantly different between the eastern and western parts of the country. In addition, 15 novel mutations have been identified.

MATERIALS AND METHODS

Patients

A total of 302 PKU or HPA patients in 290 families were analyzed after informed consent was obtained from the patients and/or their parents. In families with more than one patient, only one sibling was included. Most of the patients were identified by neonatal screening. Cofactor deficiency was excluded by the BH_4 test. Hyperphenylalaninemia was classified as classical PKU, mild PKU or HPA, by using phenylalanine (phe) pretreatment levels, phe tolerance, and 72h phe levels after phe loading adapted to previously established criteria [Güttler et al., 1993]. Accordingly, 76.8% (232/302) of the patients were classified as classical PKU, 14.2% (43/302) as mild PKU, and 9.0% (27/302) as HPA. 195 of the patients are followed at the Charité Children's Hospital in Berlin, and the remaining 107 patients are followed at the Children's Hospital in Leipzig and Jena. In Leipzig and Jena, all patients are non-immigrant Germans, mostly originating from the southeastern federal states of Saxony, Saxony-Anhalt and Thuringia. In Berlin 161 families are non-immigrant Germans, while of the other 22, 14 immigrated from Turkey and 8 from other European countries.

Laboratory Methods

Genomic DNA was isolated from peripheral leukocytes and amplified by polymerase chain reaction (PCR) using primers described previously [Zschocke et al., 1995; Dworniczak et al., 1989; DiLella et al., 1988]. In Berlin, DNA sequencing (including the promoter, the entire exonic and the flanking intronic sequences) was then performed using biotinylated amplification primers and separation of the double-stranded PCR products using Dynabeads (Dynal, Oslo, Norway) [Thein and Hinton, 1991]. Novel mutations were confirmed by allele-specific oligonucleotide hybridisation. The IVS10-11G>A mutation was identified by Dde I restriction analysis of the intron 10/exon 11/intron 11 fragment [PAH Mutation Analysis Consortium, 1996].

The samples from Jena and Leipzig were analyzed at the Leipzig Institute of Human Genetics, where PCR products were first examined by allele-specific oligonucleotide hybridisation and restriction analysis to identify common European mutations. Denaturing gradient gel electrophoresis (DGGE) was next applied, using previously described conditions [Guldberg et al., 1993]. Finally, those regions of the gene with abnormal DGGE patterns were sequenced.

RESULTS

In the 290 non-immigrant and immigrant German families, we found a total of 75 different mutations, including 15 novel mutations (Table 1).

TABLE 1. Mutation Analysis of Patients With PKU/HPA in Berlin, Jena and Leipzig

Mutations	n	%
R408W	221	38.1
IVS12+1G>A	44	7.6
IVS10-11G>A	33	5.7
R261Q	23	4.0
R158Q	19	3.3
Y414C	19	3.3
L48S	18	3.1
P281L	17	2.9
I65T	9	1.6
A104D	8	1.4
G272X	8	1.4
K274fsdel11bp	8	1.4
E390G	7	1.2
F39L	5	0.9
IVS2+5G>C	5	0.9
R68S	5	0.9
R243Q	5	0.9
R252W	5	0.9
L348V	4	0.7
IVS10-3C>T	4	0.7
A395P	4	0.7
R243X	3	0.5
A246fsdelC	3	0.5
R361X	3	0.5
IVS7+1G>A	3	0.5
IVS8+1G>A	3	0.5
M1R	2	0.3
F55fsdelT	2	0.3
F55L	2	0.3
D84Y	2	0.3
IVS4+5C>G	2	0.3
L197fsdel22bp	2	0.3
E280K	2	0.3
IVS7+5G>A	2	0.3
F299C	2	0.3
I306V	2	0.3
A309V	2	0.3
S349P	2	0.3
Y386C	2	0.3
A403V	2	0.3
Other mutations[1]	35	6.0
Unknown	31	5.3
Total	580	100

[1]Other mutations (n=1; 0.2%): Q20L, F39del, L41P, G46S, I94S, I94del, S110C, G148S, R155P, N167I, V190A, P211T, V230I, S231F, V245A, Y277D, E280-IVS7+3fsdel8bp, I283F, A300S, A309D, IVS9+1G>A, Y325C, E330D, G344V, G344R, G352fsdelG, IVS10+1G>A, Y356X, Y387H, V388M, R408Q, F410S, R413P, D415N, Ter452del5bp.

TABLE 2. Allele Frequencies of the Most Common Mutations in 276 German and 14 Turkish Families With PKU/HPA

Mutation	German families %	n	Turkish families %	n
R408W	40.1	215	0.0	0
IVS12+1G>A	8.2	44	0.0	0
IVS10-11G>A	3.0	16	57.0	16
IVS2+5G>C	0.2	1	14.5	4
L197fsdel22bp	0.0	0	7.0	2
Y386C	0.0	0	7.0	2
Others	48.5	260	14.5	4
Total	100	536	100	28

The most frequent mutations were R408W (38.1%), IVS12+1G>A (7.6%), and IVS10-11G>A (5.7%). 35 of the mutations were found on only one allele. In the Berlin group, only 1.9% (7/364) of the mutants remained unidentified after sequencing the entire coding sequence and the flanking sequences of the exon–intron boundaries. There was no significant difference in the frequencies of the mutations among the Berlin, Leipzig and Jena groups, although the diagnostic strategy resulted in 11% more unidentified mutants (24/214) in the Leipzig/Jena group.

A total of 69 different mutations were identified in the 268 independent non-immigrant German families. Except for R408W, which accounted for 40.1% of the mutant alleles, all other mutations were rare. IVS12+1G>A was the next most frequent mutation in these families, accounting for 8.2%. All other 67 mutations occurred in less than 5%. 49% (34/69) of the mutations were identified on only one allele in the non-immigrant German families. The group of the non-related immigrant Turkish families was much less heterogeneous with IVS10-11G>A accounting for 57.0% and IVS2+5G>C for 14.5% of the mutant alleles (Table 2).

We found that 29% (22/75) of the mutations were associated with mild PKU and/or HPA, but 10 of these mutations were also found in patients with classical PKU (Table 3). In one family both siblings with the same genotype (I306V/R408W) showed different clinical phenotypes, indicating the presence of genetic or non-genetic modifying factors. In the Berlin group, twelve novel mutations were identified in single patients, including nine missense mutations, two deletions and one splice-site mutation. In the Leipzig/Jena group new mutations were identified in six patients, including three missense mutations and two deletions (Table 4). Two novel mutations, in-

TABLE 3. PAH Mutations Associated With the Phenotype of Classical PKU, Mild PKU and/or HPA*

Mutation	Classic PKU n	Mild PKU n	HPA n
Q20L	–	–	1/1
F39L	3/5	1/5	1/5
L41P	–	1/1	–
L48S	7/18	8/18	3/18
F55L	–	–	2/2
I65T	8/9	1/9	–
R68S	3/6	1/6	2/6
A104D	5/8	1/8	2/8
S110C	–	–	1/1
R158Q	15/19	3/19	1/19
V190A	–	1/1	–
V230I	–	–	1/1
V245A	–	–	1/1
R252W	3/5	2/5	–
R261Q	14/23	4/23	5/23
A300S	–	–	1/1
I306V	1/3	1/3	1/3
A309V	–	2/2	–
E390G	–	4/6	2/6
A403V	–	–	4/4
F410S	–	1/1	–
Y414C	4/20	14/20	2/20

*108 patients were compound heterozygous for the mutations shown here and a severe PKU mutation; 26 patients were compound heterozygous for two of the mutations shown here; and 2 patients were homozygous for mutation A309V or E390G, respectively.

HUMAN	PAH	M	Q	L	R	E	S	Y	E	G*	F
RAT	PAH	M	Q	L	R	E	S	Y	E	G*	F
DM	PAH	M	I	R	A	E	S	F	E	G*	F
CV	PAH	–	–	–	T	D	N	–	A	G*	A
PA	PAH	–	–	–	–	E	N	Y	E	G*	F
		M1R[1]	Q20L[2]	L41P	R155P	E183Q	S231F	Y325C	E330G[3]	G344R G344V	F410S[4]

FIGURE 1. Phylogenetic conservation of PAH amino acid positions affected by the novel missense mutations. *Identical to tryptophane hydroxylase and tyrosine hydroxylase. [1]Highly conserved translation start site. [2]Exonic part of the exon 1/intron 1 splice donor consensus. [3]Iron binding site. [4]Tetramerization domain. References: OMIM Database; Dahl and Mercer, 1986; Onishi et al., 1991; Ruiz-Vázquez et al., 1996; Zhao et al., 1994. Abbreviations: DM, Drosophila melanogaster; CV, Chromobacterium violaceum; PA, Pseudomonas aeroginosa.

TABLE 4. Novel PAH Gene Mutations and Clinical Phenotype in Patients With PKU/HPA

ID	Novel mutation Amino acid	Novel mutation Nucleotide	Phylogenetic conservation[1]	Mutation in trans	Clinical phenotype	Clinical details	Special remarks
13	M1R	c.2T>G	Yes	R408W	Classical PKU	—	Abolishing the translation Initiating codon
LJ	M1R	c.2T>G	Yes	R408W	Classical PKU	Delayed diagnosis, debility	
TN	Q20L	c.59A>T	Incomplete	IVS12+1G>A	HPA	Diet: 900 mg phe/day	Results in an amino acid substitution and affects the splice consensus at the exon 1–intron 1 junction
LH	L41P	c.122T>C	Incomplete	R243Q	Mild PKU	—	Change of a neutral amino acid to a heterocyclic amino acid
SD	R155P	c.464G>C	Incomplete	R408W	Classical PKU	High phe tolerance (25 mg/kg bw/day at an age of 5 years)	Change of a basic amino acid to a heterocyclic amino acid
DD	E183Q	c.547G>C	Yes	P211T	Classical PKU	Both parents and one sister affected (mild PKU/HPA)	In cis with R408W: suspected co-segregating atypical PKU
MT	S231F	c.692C>T	Yes	K274fsdel11bp	Classical PKU	—	Change of a neutral amino acid to an aromatic amino acid
SM	Y325C	c.974A>G	Yes	L348V	Classical PKU	—	Change of an aromatic amino acid to a S-containing amino acid
14	E330D	c.990G>C	Yes	R408W	Classical PKU	—	Involved in iron building
ST	G344R	c.1030G>C	Yes	IVS12+1G>A	Classical PKU	—	Change of a neutral amino acid to a basic amino acid
Rl.a	G344V	c.1081G>T	Yes	R243Q	Classical PKU	Sibling of Rl.b	Replacing a polar amino acid with a hydrophobic amino acid
Rl.b	G344V	c.1031G>T	Yes	R243Q	Classical PKU	Growth retardation, sibling of Rl.a	
77	F410S	c.1229T>C	Yes	P281L	Mild PKU (?)	Low phe pretreatment level (10.4 mg/dl), but low phe tolerance (12 mg/kg bw/day)	Change of an aromatic amino acid to a neutral amino acid — affecting the tetramerization domain
TD	A246fsdelC	c.737delC		A403V	HPA	Vegetarian diet; sibling of TD	Frame shift of the open reading frame — premature termination of translation at codon 340 in exon 10
FD	A246fsdelC	c.737delC		A403V	HPA	Vegetarian diet; sibling of RD	
19	A246fsdelC	c.737delC		R408W	Classical PKU	—	
55	A246fsdelC	c.737delC		R408W	Classical PKU	—	
JB	E280-IVS7+3sdel8bp	c.838del8bp	Yes	R408W	Classical PKU	Dysgrammatism	Deletion of 5 base pairs at the 3′end of exon 7 and 3 base pairs at the intron 7 splice donor
60	Ter452del5bp	c.1357-1361del	Yes	L48S	Mild PKU	—	Displacing the translation stop codon to an in frame position 105 nucleotides further 3′
EF	IVS9+1G>A		Yes	R408W	Classical PKU	Initial severe dermatitis	Affecting the critical nucleotide at position +1 of the splice donor of intron 9

[1]See Figure 1.

cluding a missense mutation and a deletion, were identified in both groups.

DISCUSSION

The molecular spectrum of PAH deficiency in the eastern part of Germany is shown to be both remarkably heterogeneous and different from that in west Germany. R408W accounts for 40.1% of all mutations in the group of the non-immigrant east Germans, whereas in the studies from the western part of Germany this mutation was reported in only about 20% of the PKU alleles. In contrast, IVS12+1G>A is more frequent in the west, accounting for 11–25%, as compared to 8.2% in eastern Germany [Okano et al., 1991; Guldberg et al., 1996]. The decrease in the frequency of R408W and the increase in the frequency of IVS12+1G>A from east to west across Europe can thus also be found within Germany. On the basis of haplotype analysis, this genetic gradient has been explained by a Slavic or Balto-Slavic origin of R408W and an Anglo-Saxon origin of IVS12+1G>A [Eisensmith et al., 1995; Zschocke et al., 1997]. Therefore, it is likely that the different frequencies of the R408W and IVS12+1G>A mutations observed here can be explained by this genetic gradient across Europe.

It is interesting to note that some mutations were found to be associated with both the classical and the mild PKU/HPA phenotype (Table 3). Most of these mutations have previously been shown to result in a mild phenotype [PAH Mutation Analysis Consortium, 1996]. Phenotypic differences between patients with the same mild mutation have also been reported [Kayaalp et al., 1997; Guldberg et al., 1998], indicating that the severity of the PKU phenotype may be modified by other genetic or non-genetic factors.

The rate of unidentified mutations is low, but it depends on the strategy of analysis. The unidentified mutations are likely to be situated in the intronic regions of the PAH gene. The high degree of heterogeneity in the east German PKU patients, the low frequency of most individual mutations, and the high rate of compound heterozygotes precludes a meaningful statistical analysis of a genotype–phenotype correlation in this population. In the absence of a functional assay of enzyme activity associated with novel mutations, we used the following as parameters for the likely functional effect of the novel mutations: the phylogenetic conservation of the amino acid sequence (Fig. 1); the biochemical structure; and the clinical phenotype. According to these criteria, at least 14 of the 15 novel mutations are likely to represent bona fide mutations rather than polymorphisms. The N-terminal domain (residues 2–110) contains regulatory elements, but it is phylogenetically less conserved than the catalytically active C-terminal domain (residues 112-452) [Chehin et al., 1998]. The novel missense mutations located in the N-terminal region (Q20L, L41P) are associated with a mild phenotype, whereas the novel missense mutations located in the C-terminal region are associated with classical PKU.

M1R abolishes the translation start codon and is therefore likely to completely inactivate PAH. Q20L affects the splice donor consensus at a weakly conserved position [Aebi et al., 1986; Talerico and Berget, 1990], and it seems to be associated with an HPA phenotype. The reduction of enzyme activity may be caused by the amino acid substitution and/or by an impairment of splicing efficiency. Functional assays show that Glu 330 is involved in iron binding and that phe 410 represents the start of the tetramerization domain [Fusetti et al., 1998], indicating possible mechanisms for the effect of the novel E330D and the F410S mutations.

The family with the novel E183Q mutation with R408W in cis and P211T in trans is puzzling (see "DD" in Table 4). The index patient with classical PKU was identified by neonatal screening. Genotype analysis demonstrated the presence of all three mutations. Both of his parents are clinically healthy but exhibited the biochemical characteristics of HPA (plasma phe concentration 6.9 mg/dl and 11.6 mg/dl). The father was shown to be heterozygous for the P211T mutation, and the mother was heterozygous for the E183Q/R408W double mutation. The index patient's sister has mild PKU which was identified by neonatal screening at a time when BH4 testing was not generally performed in the former German Democratic Republic. She does not carry any of her brother's mutations. We assume that in this family PAH deficiency and atypical PKU co-segregate. Unfortunately, this family is not available for BH4 testing or further biochemical analysis. The present analysis of this family does not allow functional definition of the E183Q mutation as a bona fide mutation or a polymorphism.

The cytosine deletion A246fsdelC results in a premature translation stop codon, whereas the E280-IVS7-3fsdel8bp deletion not only shifts the reading frame of the mRNA but is also expected to affect splicing efficiency by removing the splice donor site. Both deletions are likely to result in a null phenotype because the encoded protein is C-terminally truncated, and protein synthesis is likely to be reduced to low levels due to degradation of the mRNA by a mechanism termed *nonsense mediated decay* [Hentze and Kulozik, 1999]. The deletion Ter452del5bp affects the translation termination codon and causes an elongation of the polypeptide by 35 amino acids. There is no precedent for a similar mutation of the PAH gene, but Ter mutations of other genes have been reported to impair the stability of the affected mRNA [Weiss and Liebhaber, 1994]. The novel splicing mutation IVS9+1G>A affects the highly conserved GT donor site [Aebi et al., 1986; Talerico and Berget, 1990], and is thus likely to completely abolish gene expression.

In summary, the molecular analysis of PKU/HPA in the eastern part of Germany has revealed a heterogeneous spectrum of mutations which is significantly different from the western part of the country. Additionally, fifteen novel mutations were identified, including eleven missense mutations, three deletions and one splicing mutation.

REFERENCES

Aebi M, Hornig H, Padgett RA, Reiser J, Weissmann C. 1986. Sequence requirements for splicing of higher eukaryotic nuclear pre-mRNA. Cell 47:555–565.

Baranovskaya S, Shevtsov S, Maksimova S, Kuzmin A, Schwartz E. 1996. The mutations and VNTRs in the phenylalanine hydroxylase gene of phenylketonuria in St Petersburg. J Inher Metab Dis 19:705.

Chehin R, Thorolfsson M, Knappskog PM, Martinez M, Flatmark T, Arrondo JLR, Muga A. 1998. Domain structure and stability of human phenylalanine hydroxylase inferred from infrared spectroscopy. FEBS Letters 422:225–230.

Dahl H-HM, Mercer JFB. 1986. Isolation and sequence of a cDNA clone which contains the complete coding region of rat phenylalanine hydroxylase: structural homology with tyrosine hydroxylase, glucocorticoid regulation, and use of alternate polyadenylation sites. J Biol Chem 261:4148–4153.

Desviat LR, Pérez B, Ugarte M. 1997. Phenylketonuria in Spanish gypsies: prevalence of the IVS10nt546 mutation on haplotype 34. Hum Mutat 9:66–68.

DiLella AG, Huang WM, Woo SL. 1988. Screening for phenylketonuria mutations by DNA amplification with the polymerase chain reaction. Lancet 1:497–499.

Dworniczak B, Aulehla-Scholz C, Horst J. 1989. Phenylketonuria: detection of a frequent haplotype 4 allele mutation. Hum Genet 84:95–96.

Eisensmith RC, Goltsov AA, O'Neill CO, Tyfield LA, Schwartz EI, Kuzmin AI, Baranovskaya SS, Tsukerman GL, Treacy E, Scriver CR, Güttler F, Guldbergf P, Eiken HG, Apold J, Svensson E, Naughten E, Cahalane SF, Crooke DT, Cockburn F, Woo SLC. 1995. Recurrence of the R408W mutation in the phenylalanine hydroxylase locus in Europeans. Am J Hum Genet 56:278–286.

Fusetti F, Erlandsen H, Flatmark T, Stevens RC. 1998. Structure of tetrameric human phenylalanine hydroxylase and its implications for phenylketonuria. J Biol Chem 27:16962–16967.

Guldberg P, Henriksen KF, Güttler F. 1993. Molecular analysis of phenylketonuria in Denmark: 99% of the mutations detected by denaturing gradient gel electrophoresis. Genomics 17:141–146.

Guldberg P, Mallmann R, Henriksen KF, Güttler F. 1996. Phenylalanine hydroxylase deficiency in a population in Germany: mutation profile and nine novel mutations. Hum Mutat 8:276–279.

Guldberg P, Rey F, Zschocke J, Romano V, Francois B, Michiels L, Ullrich K, Hoffmann GF, Burgard P, Schmidt H, Meli C, Riva E, Dianzani I, Ponzone A, Rey J, Güttler F. 1998. A European multicenter study of phenylalanine hydroxylase deficiency: classification of 105 mutations and a general system for genotype based prediction of metabolic phenotype. Am J Hum Genet 63:71–79.

Güttler F, Guldberg KF, Henriksen KF, Mikkelsen I, Olsen B, Lou H. 1993. Molecular basis for the phenotypical diversity of phenylketonuria and related hyperphenylalaninemias. J Inher Metab Dis 16:602.

Guzzetta V, Bonapace G, Dianzani I, Parenti G, Lecora M, Giannattasio S, Concolino D, Strisciuglio P, Sebastio G, Andria G. 1997. Phenylketonuria in Italy: distinct distribution pattern of three mutations of the phenylalanine hydroxylase gene. J Inher Metab Dis 20:619–624.

Hentze MW, Kulozik AE. 1999. A perfect message: RNA surveillance in humans, animals and yeast. Cell 96:307–310.

Kayaalp E, Treacy E, Waters PJ, Byck S, Nowacki P, Scriver CR. 1997. Human phenylalanine hydroxylase mutations and hyperphenylalaninemia phenotypes: a metanalysis of genotype–phenotype correlations. Am J Hum Genet 61:1309–1317.

Kozak L, Blazkova M, Kuhrova V, Pijackova A, Ruzickova S, St'astna S. 1997. Mutation and haplotype analysis of phenylalanine hydroxylase alleles in classical PKU patients from the Czech Republic: identification of four novel mutations. J Med Genet 34:893–898.

Nowacki PM, Byck S, Prevost L, Scriver CR. 1998. PAH Mutation Analysis Consortium Database 1997: prototype for relational locus-specific mutation databases. Nucleic Acids Res 26:220–225.

Okano Y, Eisensmith RC, Güttler F, Lichter-Konecki U, Konecki DS, Trefz FK, Dasovich M, Wang T, Henriksen K, Lou H, Woo SLC. 1991. Molecular basis of phenotypic heterogeneity in phenylketonuria. N Engl J Med 324:1232–1238.

Onishi A, Liotta LJ, Benkovic SJ. 1991. Cloning and expression of chromobacterium violaceum phenylalanine hydroxylase in Escherichia coli and comparison of amino acid sequence with mammalian aromatic amino acid hydroxylases. J Biol Chem 266:18454–18459.

Özalp I, Coskun T, Özgüç M, Tokath A, Yalaz K, Vanh L, Yilmaz E, Erbay A. 1994. Genetic and neurological evaluation of untreated and late treated pateints with phenylketonuria. J Inher Metab Dis 17:371.

PAH Mutation Analysis Database. 1996. Waters P, editor. Accessible via the Internet (at: http://www.mcgill.ca/pahdb).

Pérez B, Desviat LR, Ugarte M. 1997. Analysis of the phenylalanine hydroxylase gene in the Spanish population: mutation profile and association with intragenic polymorphic markers. Am J Hum Genet 60:95–102.

Ruiz-Vázquez P, Moulard M, Silva FJ. 1996. Structure of the phenylalanine hydroxylase gene in Drosophila melanogaster and evidence of alternative promoter usage. Biochem Biophys Res Comm 225:238–242.

Schuler A, Somogyi Cs, Máté M, Pataki L, Törös I, Woo SLC, Eisensmith RC, Fekete G. 1994. Cognitive development related to metabolic phenotype and mutation genotype in 25 Hungarian patients with phenylketonuria. J Inher Metab Dis 17:372.

Scriver CR, Waters PF, Sarkissian C, Ryan S, Prevost L, Cote D, Novak J, Teebi S, Nowacki PM. 2000. PAHdb: a locus-specific knowledgebase. Hum Mutat 15:99–104.

Svensson E, von Döbeln U, Eisensmith R, Hagenfeldt L, Woo SLC. 1993. Relation between genotype and phenotype in Swedish phenylketonuria and hyperphenylalninemia patients. Eur J Pediatr 152:132–139.

Talerico M, Berget SM. 1990. Effect of 5′ splice site mutations on splicing of the preceding intron. Mol Cell Biol 10:6299–6305.

Thein SL, Hinton J. 1991. A simple and rapid method of direct sequencing using Dynabeads. Br J Haematol 79:113–115.

Weiss IM, Liebhaber SA. 1994. Erythroid cell-specific determinants of α-globin mRNA stability. Mol Cell Biol 14:8123–8132.

Zhao G, Xia T, Song J, Jensen RA. 1994. Pseudomonas aeroginosa possesses homologues of mammalian phenylalanine hydroxylase and 4 alpha-carbinolamine dehydratase/DCOH as part of a three-component gene cluster. Proc Natl Acad Sci USA 91:1366–1370.

Zschocke J, Graham CA, Carson DJ, Nevin NC. 1995. Phenylketonuria mutation analysis in Northern Ireland: a rapid stepwise approach. Am J Hum Genet 57:1311–1317.

Zschocke J, Mallory JP, Eiken HG, Nevin NC. 1997. Phenylketonuria and the peoples of Northern Ireland. Hum Genet 100:189–194.

Zygulska M, Eigel A, Dworniczak B, Sutkowska A, Pietrzyk JJ, Horst J. 1991. Phenylketonuria in Poland: 66% of PKU alleles are caused by three mutations. Hum Genet 88:91–94.

2.2. PUBLIKATION 2: Hennermann JB, Roloff S, Gellermann J, Vollmer I, Windt E, Vetter B, Plöckinger U, Mönch E, Querfeld U. Chronic Kidney Disease in Adolescent and Adult Patients with Phenylketonuria. 2013. J Inherit Metab Dis 36:747–756. DOI 10.1007/s10545-012-9548-0

Reprinted from: Journal of Inherited Metabolic Disease 2013, Volume 36 (5), page 747-56, with permission from SSIEM and Springer Science + Business Media Dordrecht 2012, provided by Springer, Head of Rights and Permissions

Bei PKU-Patienten erfolgt der Hauptteil der Proteinzufuhr, nämlich 75-95% der Gesamt-Proteinzufuhr, über die Gabe des Phe-freien synthetischen Aminosäurengemisches. Aminosäurengemische bestehen aus Mono-Aminosäuren, die schneller metabolisiert werden als Aminosäuren, die aus natürlichem Protein stammen (Mönch et al. 1996). Es ist außerdem bekannt, dass die Proteinzufuhr einen relevanten Einfluss auf die Nierenfunktion hat (Brenner et al. 1982; King und Levey 1993). Wir untersuchten daher den Einfluss der Phe-bilanzierten Diät auf die Nierenfunktion von adoleszenten und erwachsenen Patienten mit PKU. Bei 67 Patienten im Alter zwischen 15-43 Jahren wurden die glomeruläre Filtrationsrate (GFR) sowie der effektive renale Plasmafluss mittels Isotopen-Clearance (^{51}Cr-EDTA, ^{123}J-Hippuran), die Retentionsparameter, die Protein- und Elektrolyt-Ausscheidung im Urin, eine Nierenultraschalluntersuchung und eine 24-Stunden-Blutdruckmessung durchgeführt.

Zum Zeitpunkt der Untersuchung lag die Gesamtproteinzufuhr der untersuchten PKU-Patienten bei 0.96 ± 0.23 g/kg KG/Tag. 24% der Patienten waren übergewichtig (BMI 25-30 kg/m²), 13% der Patienten adipös (BMI >30 kg/m²). Eine arterielle Hypertonie zeigte sich bei 23% der Patienten, zudem fehlte bei 41% der Patienten der physiologische nächtliche Blutdruck-Abfall. Die Blutdruckwerte waren nicht mit GFR, Proteinzufuhr oder Proteinurie assoziiert, jedoch signifikant mit dem BMI. 19% der Patienten wiesen eine Erniedrigung der GFR auf, 31% eine Proteinurie, 7% eine Mikroalbuminurie und 23% eine Hyperkalziurie. Mit steigender Proteinzufuhr fiel die GFR signifikant ab, bezogen auf die aktuelle Gesamtprotein-Zufuhr, die aktuelle Zufuhr an synthetischem Eiweiß und die lebenslange Proteinzufuhr. Auch die Proteinurie war signifikant mit steigender Proteinzufuhr assoziiert. Die erhöhte Kalziumausscheidung war mit der aktuellen Proteinzufuhr, insbesondere der Zufuhr an synthetischem Eiweiß assoziiert; es gab jedoch keinen Einfluss der lebenslangen Proteinzufuhr auf die Kalziumausscheidung. Mittels multivarianter Regressionsanalyse zeigten sich lediglich Proteinurie und aktuelle Gesamt-Proteinzufuhr als unabhängige Prädiktoren der GFR mittels Isotopen-Clearance (p <0,005). Der Vergleich der Patientengruppe mit eingeschränkter GFR mit der Patientengruppe mit normaler GFR erbrachte ebenfalls signifikante Unterschiede bezüglich Proteinurie und lebenslanger Proteinzufuhr (s. Tabelle 3). Eine Assoziation mit den unterschiedlichen Genotypen der Patienten und der Nierenfunktion oder der arteriellen Hypertonie ergab sich nicht.

Keiner der Patienten wies eine Hyperaminoazidurie auf. Die Phe-Konzentration im Urin war auf 0,713 ± 0,375 mmol/g Kreatinin erhöht und korrelierte signifikant mit aktuellen sowie lebenslangen Phe-Plasmakonzentrationen, GFR, Proteinurie, und systolischem Blutdruck. Die Phe-Plasmakonzentration war zum Zeitpunkt der Untersuchung 796 ± 317 µmol/L (aktuelle Empfehlungen für Patienten >15 Jahre 40-1200 µmol/L; Burgard et al. 1999) und lag nur bei 4 von 67 Patienten oberhalb des therapeutischen Zielbereiches. Aktuelle oder lebenslange Phe-Plasmakonzentrationen korrelierten nicht mit GFR, Proteinurie oder Blutdruck.

Anhand dieser Daten konnten wir erstmals nachweisen, dass PKU-Patienten unter der Phe-bilanzierten Diät eine chronische Nierenerkrankung (eingeschränkte Nierenfunktion, Proteinurie) sowie eine arterielle Hypertonie entwickeln können.

Tabelle 3: Alter, BMI, Protein-Zufuhr, Protein- Ausscheidung, Kalzium-Ausscheidung sowie systolischer Blutdruck in PKU-Patienten mit verminderter und mit normaler GFR

GFR	Anzahl der Patienten	GFR (ml/min/1,73m²)	Alter (Jahre)[1]	BMI (kg/m²)[1]	Zufuhr natürliches Protein (g/kg/die)[1]	Zufuhr synthet. Protein (g/kg/die)[1]	Zufuhr Gesamt Protein (g/kg/die)[1]	Lebenslange Diät* (Jahre)[2]	Urin-Protein (g/g Krea)[2]	Urin-Kalzium (g/g Krea)[1]	Systolischer Blutdruck (mm/Hg)[1]
vermindert	11	87 ± 8,5 (64 - 94)	23,2 ± 4,3	24,0 ± 4,5	0,31 ± 0,24	0,65 ± 0,42	0,96 ± 0,27	20 ± 2,7	150 ± 79	0,15 ± 0,16	125 ± 13
normal	48	111 ± 13,1 (95 - 149)	23,9 ± 6,8	23,7 ± 4,0	0,31 ± 0,19	0,67 ± 0,35	0,97 ± 0,23	15 ± 6,0	135 ± 252	0,16 ± 0,07	125 ± 10

Angabe der Daten in Mittelwert ± Standardabweichung

[1] nicht signifikant; [2] p = 0,03

*Lebenslange Diät: kumulative Anzahl der Jahre, in denen die tägliche Proteinzufuhr die Empfehlungen der Deutschen Gesellschaft für Ernährung von 1985 überschritt (DGE Empfehlung 1985).

Obwohl sich die aktuelle Protein-Zufuhr bei Patienten mit verminderter und normaler GFR nicht unterschied, war die kumulative Anzahl der Jahre, in denen die tägliche Proteinzufuhr die Empfehlungen der Deutschen Gesellschaft für Ernährung von 1985 überschritt, bei Patienten mit verminderter GFR signifikant höher als bei Patienten mit normaler GFR. Zudem war die Proteinausscheidung bei Patienten mit verminderter GFR signifikant höher als bei Patienten mit normaler GFR. Unterschiede bezüglich des Alters, des BMI, der Kalziumausscheidung sowie des Blutdrucks ergaben sich bei den beiden Patientengruppen nicht.

ORIGINAL ARTICLE

Chronic kidney disease in adolescent and adult patients with phenylketonuria

Julia B. Hennermann · Sylvia Roloff · Jutta Gellermann · Ilka Vollmer · Elke Windt · Barbara Vetter · Ursula Plöckinger · Eberhard Mönch · Uwe Querfeld

Received: 19 March 2012 / Revised: 13 September 2012 / Accepted: 4 October 2012 / Published online: 9 November 2012
© SSIEM and Springer Science+Business Media Dordrecht 2012

Communicated by: Eva Morava

Eberhard Mönch and Uwe Querfeld both authors contributed equally to the study.

Electronic supplementary material The online version of this article (doi:10.1007/s10545-012-9548-0) contains supplementary material, which is available to authorized users.

J. B. Hennermann (✉) · S. Roloff
Department of Pediatric Endocrinology, Gastroenterology and Metabolic Diseases, Charité Universitätsmedizin Berlin, Augustenburger Platz 1,
13353 Berlin, Germany
e-mail: julia.hennermann@charite.de

J. Gellermann · I. Vollmer · U. Querfeld
Department of Pediatric Nephrology, Charité Universitätsmedizin Berlin,
Berlin, Germany

E. Windt
Department of Neuropediatrics, Charite Universitätsmedizin Berlin,
Berlin, Germany

B. Vetter
Department of Pediatric Molecular Medicine,
Charité Universitätsmedizin Berlin,
Augustenburger Platz 1,
13353 Berlin, Germany

U. Plöckinger · E. Mönch
Department of Hepatology and Gastroenterology, Charité Universitätsmedizin Berlin,
Berlin, Germany

Abstract

Objectives A lifelong phenylalanine-restricted diet with supplementation of a phenylalanine-free amino acid formula is recommended in patients with phenylketonuria (PKU). The effect of a long-term PKU diet on renal function and blood pressure has not been investigated yet.

Design We analyzed renal function in 67 patients with PKU, aged 15–43 years, by measuring glomerular filtration rate (GFR) and effective renal plasma flow by isotope clearance (^{51}Cr-EDTA, ^{123}J-Hippuran), estimated GFR, blood retention parameters, urinary protein and electrolyte excretion. Renal ultrasound and 24 h ambulatory blood pressure monitoring were performed additionally. Patients were divided into three groups according to their: 1) current diet (CD), i.e., daily protein intake: I_{CD} <0.8 g/kg, II_{CD} 0.8–1.04 g/kg, III_{CD} >1.04 g/kg; 2) life-long diet time (LDT), i.e., cumulative years of life in which daily protein intake exceeded dietary recommendations: I_{LDT} <15 years, II_{LDT} 15–19 years, III_{LDT} >19 years.

Results GFR was decreased in 19 % of the patients. With increasing protein intake, GFR decreased significantly (I_{CD} 111 ml/min; II_{CD} 105 ml/min; III_{CD} 99 ml/min. I_{LDT} 112 ml/min; II_{LDT} 103 ml/min; III_{LDT} 99 ml/min). Proteinuria was detected in 31 %, microalbuminuria in 7 %, and hypercalciuria in 23 % of the patients. 23 % of the patients had arterial hypertension, and 41 % revealed a nocturnal non-dipping status.

Conclusions In patients with PKU on a lifelong diet we could detect impaired renal function in 19 %, proteinuria in 31 %, and arterial hypertension in 23 %. Thus, chronic kidney disease may develop in PKU patients, and routine renal function tests should be performed during long-term follow-up.

Abbreviations

AA	Amino acids
ABPM	Ambulatory blood pressure monitoring
BMI	Body mass index
BP	Blood pressure
CD	Current diet

CKD	Chronic kidney disease
eGFR	Estimated glomerular filtration rate
ERPF	Effective renal plasma flow
GFR	Glomerular filtration rate
LDT	Life-long diet time
PAH	Phenylalanine hydroxylase
Phe	Phenylalanine
PKU	Phenylketonuria
RDA	Recommended daily allowance

Introduction

Phenylketonuria (PKU, MIM 261600) is a rare autosomal recessive inborn error of metabolism caused by phenylalanine-4-hydroxylase (PAH, EC 1.14.16.1) deficiency (Scriver and Kaufman 2001). In untreated children, PKU results in severe neurological impairment with mental retardation, seizures, and behavioral disorders. Normal mental and motor activity skills can be achieved by early institution of a phenylalanine (Phe)-restricted diet consisting of a strong restriction of natural protein intake and substitution with a Phe-free L-amino acid (AA) formula (Scriver and Kaufman 2001). The Phe-restricted diet consists of foods with low protein content, e.g., vegetables, fruits and special low-protein food products. Most of the protein supply in PKU patients, e.g., 75–95 % of the whole protein intake, derives from the prescribed Phe-free AA formula (Mönch et al 1996). The allowed amount of the daily natural protein intake is dependent on the individual residual PAH enzyme activity corresponding to the severity of the disease. At the current state of knowledge, diet is recommended to be kept life-long.

To prevent a nutritional deficiency in essential AA, patients with PKU receive high amounts of the AA formula (Krauch et al 1996). Thus, protein intake in patients with PKU almost entirely consists of the AA formula, and often exceeds the current recommended daily allowance (RDA) for the general population, especially during the first years of life (D-A-CH Empfehlung 2000; Acosta et al 1998; Arnold et al 2002; Hoeksma et al 2005). AA formulas consist of synthetic mono AA, which have a lower biological efficacy than natural protein. The intake of the synthetic AA leads to peak plasma AA concentrations shortly after ingestion resulting in a high renal acid load (Mönch et al 1996; Manz et al 1977). This is in marked contrast to the stable plasma AA concentrations after the intake of intact natural protein (Gropper et al 1993).

Dietary protein is a well known modulator of kidney function (Brenner et al 1982; King and Levey 1993). The hyperfiltration theory suggests that protein consumption acutely results in an increase of renal plasma flow and glomerular filtration rate (GFR), leading to hyperfiltration and hypertension, thus resulting in chronic glomerular injury, fibrosis and mesangial cell proliferation (Bernstein et al 2007; Brenner et al 1996). In animal experiments, a high protein diet resulted in renal and glomerular enlargement, collagen deposition and tubulointerstitial infiltration, leading to cortical fibrosis and glomerulosclerosis (Jia et al 2010). In adult patients with chronic kidney disease (CKD), a low protein diet has been recommended to delay the progression of renal failure (Brenner et al 1982; Fouque and Aparicio 2007; Schena 2011).

Patients with PKU have to keep a life-long Phe-restricted diet, but it is unknown whether the relatively high total protein intake with the high proportion of synthetic AA may have an effect on renal function. We have therefore investigated the effect of the PKU diet on renal structure, function and blood pressure (BP) in adolescent and adult patients with PAH deficiency.

Study population and methods

Study population

Eighty patients with PKU treated in the metabolic unit of the Department of Pediatrics at the Charité Berlin were eligible for this cross-sectional study evaluating clinical and biochemical data, ultrasound studies, renal function, 24-h ambulatory blood pressure monitoring (ABPM), and dietary history. Exclusion criteria were: age <15 years, pregnancy or breastfeeding. Of a total of these 80 patients, 13 refused participation completely and 28 patients refused participation in some parts of the study. Therefore, of the 67 patients participating in the study, ultrasound was performed in 61 patients, ABPM in 44 patients and radioisotope clearance studies in 59 patients. Informed consent was obtained from all patients and/or their parents.

The median age of the patients was 24 years (15–43 years) with 38 females and 29 males. According to established criteria (Guldberg et al 1998; Güttler and Guldberg 1994), 60 % of the patients were classified as classic PKU ($n=40$), 37 % as mild PKU ($n=25$) and 3 % as hyperphenylalaninemia ($n=2$). Fifty-eight patients were diagnosed by newborn screening, nine patients were diagnosed by selective screening at a median age of 42 months (3–171 months). In total, we collected data of cumulative 1600 patient-years.

Chart review showed that dietary treatment had been started in all patients immediately after diagnosis of PKU. At the time of examination, 82 % of the patients ($n=55$) kept a Phe-restricted diet with supplementation of a Phe-free AA formula, 3 % ($n=2$) kept a diet low in natural protein without additional AA formula, and 15 % ($n=10$) had stopped adhering to the diet. Protein intake was calculated regularly by three-day-dietary-protocols. At the time of examination AA formula was applied thrice a day (AA formulas and hydrolysates supplemented in the patients are shown in Supplementary Table 1).

Methods

Clinical examination including body mass index (BMI) was performed in every patient. According to the World Health Organization "overweight" was defined as a BMI equal to or more than 25, and "obesity" as a BMI equal to or more than 30. ABPM was performed by using Model 90207(−32), Spacelabs Medical (USA). Arterial hypertension was defined according to established criteria as a daytime average above systolic 135 mmHg and/or systolic 85 mmHg (Parati and Pickering 2009; O'Brien et al 2005; Wühl et al 2002). A decrease of systolic BP during nocturnal time by ≥10 % of the diurnal BP was defined as a "dipper", a decrease of <10 % as a "non-dipper" (Kastarinen et al 2010). In three patients without nocturnal sleeping phase during ABPM, "dipping"-/"non-dipping"-status was not discriminated. Renal ultrasound was performed with a 50/60 Hz transducer (Sonoline Antares, Siemens, Germany).

Laboratory analysis was performed in the fasting state in all patients and included the determination of serum creatinine, urea, uric acid, cystatin C, blood gases, electrolytes, total protein, albumin, vitamin D status and parathormone. Excretion of creatinine, protein, albumin, alpha-1-microglobuline, immunglobulin G, glucose, and electrolytes was analyzed in a 24-h urine collection. AA in plasma and urine were measured by cation exchange chromatography (Biotronic/Eppendorf). Plasma Phe was analyzed regularly in all study patients, according to the German recommendations for the treatment in PKU (Burgard et al 1999).

Renal function was determined by radio-isotope clearance: 80 kBq ^{51}Cr-EDTA/kg and 15 kBq ^{123}J-Hippuran/kg were simultaneously applied intravenously, and measured 30 min after application in a 2.0 ml plasma sample. ^{51}Cr-EDTA clearance was used to evaluate GFR, ^{123}J-Hippuran clearance to evaluate effective renal plasma flow (ERPF), and the ratio of ^{51}Cr-EDTA/^{123}J-Hippuran clearances to evaluate the filtration fraction (Hüseman et al 1999). Upper and lower cut off levels of GFR and ERPF were defined as ±2 SD. Additional informed consent for performing radio-isotope clearance was obtained from all patients and/or their parents.

The estimated GFR (eGFR) was calculated using the formula of Schwartz for adolescent patients ≤16 years ($n=$ 6) and the "modification of diet in renal disease" (MDRD) formula for adult patients ($n=61$) (Kooman 2009; Schwartz et al 2009; Staples et al 2010). Urinary creatinine clearance was not evaluated, since inaccuracy of sampling might have resulted in a falsely low estimation of GFR.

PAH genotype was determined in 60 patients, as previously described (Hennermann et al 2000). According to their genotype patients were classified into two different groups. Group 1: patients with two null mutations, corresponding to a complete loss of residual PAH activity; group 2: patients with at least one putative milder mutation, corresponding to a certain residual PAH activity. In three patients only one mutation was identified; they were not included in any group.

Statistics

For statistic analyses PASW Statistics, Version 18.0, was used. Differences between patients groups were analyzed by non-parametric tests, the Mann-Whitney-test, and the Jonckheere-Terpstra test. Significance of correlations of variables was tested with the Spearman-Rho-correlation coefficient. Multiple forward stepwise regression analysis was performed to analyze the significance of effects of several variables on the outcome variable, GFR measured by isotope clearance.

Results

Protein intake

Median current total protein intake in all 67 PKU patients was 0.96±0.23 g/kg/day. Current total protein intake was 1.01±0.23 g/kg/day in patients on a Phe-restricted diet with AA formula ($n=55$), 0.57±0.01 g/kg/day in patients on a low protein diet without AA formula ($n=2$), and 0.75± 0.00 g/kg/day in patients off PKU diet ($n=10$).

According to their dietary protein intake, patients were divided into three groups: according to the amount of their *current diet* (CD), and according to their *life-long diet time* (LDT). CD was determined by the amount of total daily protein intake and daily AA intake (Table 1). LDT was determined by the number of cumulative years of life in which the daily protein intake has exceeded German RDA of 1985 (DGE Empfehlung 1985) (Table 2).

Clinical examination

Clinical examinations revealed no significant abnormalities in any patient. Median BMI was 23.9±4.8 kg/m^2 and was increased in 25/67 patients (37.3 %). Sixteen patients (23.9 %) were overweight, nine patients were obese (13.4 %). There was an inverse correlation between BMI and actual total and synthetic protein intake ($p=0.000$; $r=-0.470$, $r=-0.421$, respectively). None of the patients was suffering from any other

Table 1 Classification of PKU patients according to their actual protein intake (CD)

Current total protein intake and current synthetic protein intake are indicated in mean with minimum and maximum.

Group	Number of patients	Current total protein intake (g/kg/day)	Current AA intake (g synthetic protein intake/kg/day)
I-CD	21	0.75 (0.56–0.79)	0 (0–0.57)
II-CD	22	0.90 (0.80–1.04)	0.70 (0.58–0.79)
III-CD	22	1.14 (1.05–1.67)	0.94 (0.80–1.45)

inborn error of metabolism or from insulin dependent or non-insulin dependent diabetes.

Renal ultrasound

Renal ultrasound revealed bilateral nephrocalcinosis in 1/61 patient, associated with increased calcium excretion. Increased renal echogenity was found in 4/61 patients (6.6 %), associated with arterial hypertension and increased calcium excretion in 3/4. None of these patients received calcium supplementation. One patient showed unilateral polycystic changes, one patient a renal position abnormality. The size of both kidneys was within normal range with a mean size of 10.7±0.75 cm (left), and 10.4±0.78 cm (right), respectively, and correlated significantly with serum creatinine ($p=0.041$).

Hypertension

Mean 24-h systolic BP was 127.0±14.1 mmHg (105–182 mmHg), diastolic BP 77.6±9.6 mmHg (58–118 mmHg), and MAD 93.4±10.4 mmHg (73–138 mmHg). Arterial hypertension was diagnosed in 22.7 % of the patients (10/44). 41 % of the patients (17/41) revealed a nocturnal non-dipping status. Neither arterial pressure nor dipping status were correlated with GFR, eGFR, protein intake (CD, LDT), or proteinuria. There was a significant correlation of all BP parameters with BMI ($p=0.000$; $r=0.510$).

GFR

GFR measured by ^{51}Cr-EDTA was 107±15.5 ml/min/1.73 m² (range 64–149; norm 95–161). GFR was decreased in 18.6 % of the patients ($n=11$) and normal in 81.4 % of the patients ($n=48$). ERPF measured by ^{123}J-Hippuran was 707±159 ml/min/1.73 m² (range 426–1197; norm 515–916), and revealed an increase corresponding to hyperfiltration in four patients (6.8 %), a decrease in five patients (8.5 %), and normal values in 50 patients (84.7 %). ERPF correlated significantly with GFR ($p=0.000$; $r=0.512$). Filtration fraction was increased in five patients (8.5 %) and normal in 54 patients (91.5 %). GFR decreased significantly with increasing protein intake, both was correlated with CD and LDT (Figs. 1, 2, and 3). GFR was associated with BMI ($p=0.025$; $r=0.295$); in contrast, there was no correlation of GFR with the patient's age. Neither ERPF nor filtration fraction were correlated with CD or LDT. Data of patients with diminished GFR are included in Supplementary Table 2.

The eGFR correlated significantly with ^{51}Cr-EDTA (Fig. 4). eGFR was 108±18.1 ml/min/1.73 m² (range 74–157; norm 90–160). eGFR was decreased in 10.4 % of the patients ($n=7$) and normal in 89.6 % of the patients ($n=60$). The eGFR did not correlate with CD, LDT or BMI.

By multiple forward stepwise regression analysis, only proteinuria and the current total protein intake were independent predictors of the GFR estimated by isotope clearance ($p<0.005$; $r^2=0.201$).

Table 2 Classification of PKU patients according to their life-long protein intake (LDT)

Group	Number of patients	Number of years exceeding protein intake
I-LDT	19	12 (4–14)
II-LDT	17	17 (15–19)
III-LDT	19	22 (20–34)

Indicated are the number of years in which the total protein intake in PKU patients exceeded the German RDA from 1985 (DGE Empfehlung 1985) Values are indicated in mean with minimum and maximum

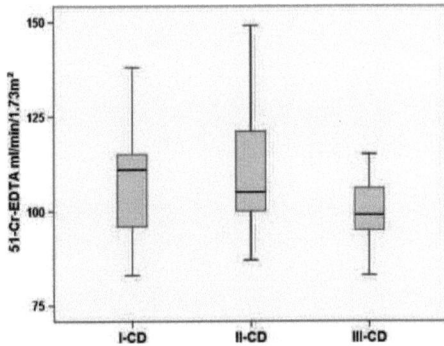

Fig. 1 ^{51}Cr-EDTA related to current total protein intake ^{51}Cr-EDTA was measured in 59 patients. Median ^{51}Cr-EDTA was 111 ml/min in the group with the lowest total protein intake (I-CD), 105 ml/min in the group with the medium total protein intake (II-CD), and 99 ml/min in the group with the highest total protein intake (III-CD). The correlation of ^{51}Cr-EDTA with current total protein intake was significant ($p=0.008$; $r=0.341$)

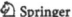

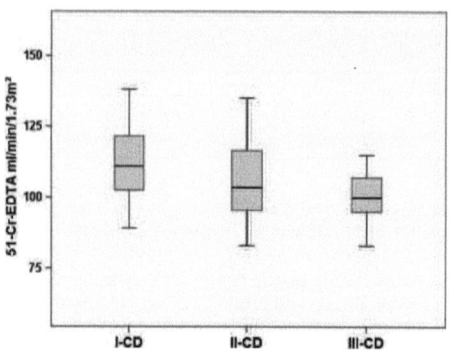

Fig. 2 ^{51}Cr-EDTA related to current AA intake (synthetic protein intake) ^{51}Cr-EDTA was measured in 59 patients. Median ^{51}Cr-EDTA was 111 ml/min in the group with the lowest AA intake (I-CD), 105 ml/min in the group with the medium AA intake (II-CD), and 100 ml/min in the group with the highest AA intake (III-CD). The correlation of ^{51}Cr-EDTA with current AA intake was significant ($p=0.011$; $r=-0.331$)

Creatinine and cystatin C serum concentrations were within normal ranges in all patients. There was a significant correlation between serum creatinine and ^{51}Cr-EDTA ($p=0.000$; $r=0.519$). Both, creatinine and cystatin C, increased non-significantly with increasing protein consumption.

Proteinuria and Phe excretion

Mean serum levels of protein and albumin were within normal ranges. Proteinuria, defined as a protein excretion

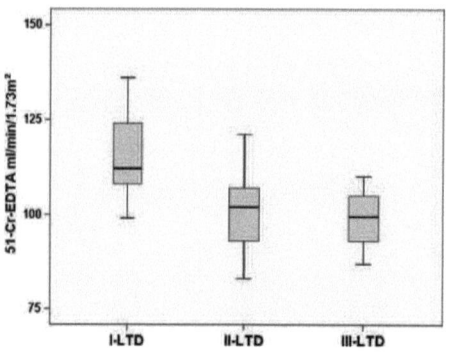

Fig. 3 ^{51}Cr-EDTA related to life-long-diet ^{51}Cr-EDTA was measured in 59 patients. Median ^{51}Cr-EDTA was 112 ml/min in the group with the lowest life-long protein intake (I-LDT), 103 ml/min in the group with the medium life-long protein intake (II-LDT), and 99 ml/min in the group with the highest life-long protein intake (III-LDT). The correlation of ^{51}Cr-EDTA with life-long-diet was significant ($p=0.003$; $r=-0.410$)

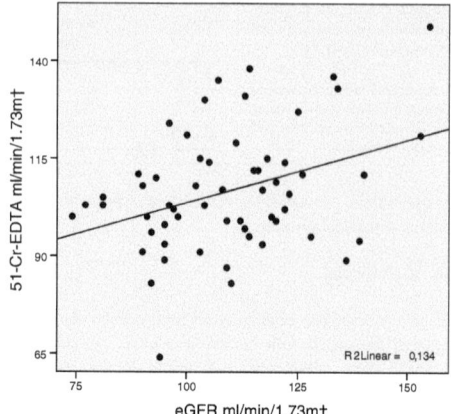

Fig. 4 ^{51}Cr-EDTA related to eGFR ^{51}Cr-EDTA was measured in 59 patients, eGFR in 67 patients. The correlation of ^{51}Cr-EDTA and eGFR was significant ($p=0.029$; $r=0.285$)

of >150 mg/24 h (Guy et al 2009), was found in 19/62 patients (30.6 %). Microalbuminuria, defined as an albumin excretion of 30–300 mg/g creatinine (Blecker et al 2011), was detected in 4/62 patients (6.5 %). Proteinuria was not correlated to BMI. The excretion of alpha-1-microglobulin was increased in one patient (18.3 mg/g creatinine), the excretion of immunglobulin G in two patients (maximum 25.1 mg/g creatinine).

Urinary AA analysis revealed no hyperaminoaciduria in any patient. Urinary Phe concentrations were increased to 0.713±0.375 mmol/g creatinine (range 0.087–2.429; norm <0.19) and correlated significantly with actual and life-long Phe plasma concentrations ($p=0.000$, $p=0.001$; $r=0.727$, $r=0.488$, respectively). Urinary Phe excretion correlated significantly with GFR ($p=0.011$; $r=0.332$), proteinuria ($p=0.007$; $r=0.338$), and systolic BP ($p=0.040$; $r=0.311$). Actual Phe plasma levels were 796± 317 μmol/L (range 169–2,143; recommendations for PKU patients >15 years 40–1,200) and exceeded actual German recommendations in only 4/67 patients. However, actual or life-long plasma Phe concentrations did not correlate with GFR, eGFR, proteinuria, or BP.

Calcium, phosphate, hypercalciuria and vitamin D

Serum calcium was slightly increased in 3/61 patients (4.9 %), and serum phosphate was decreased in 3/59 patients (5.1 %). Calcium excretion was 0.17±0.09 g/g creatinine (range 0.04–0.54; norm <0.2) and was increased in 22.7 % of the patients (15/66). Renal tubular reabsorption of phosphate (TmP/GFR) was within the normal range (0.96±0.27 mmol/L; norm 0.6–1.7 mmol/L). In only two patients, both, calcium and phosphate excretion were increased. The serum calcium phosphate product was normal in all patients. An increase in calcium excretion was significantly associated with CD, mainly with actual synthetic AA intake (Fig. 5), but there was no correlation to LDT. Phosphate reabsorption was not correlated to CD or LDT. Venous blood gas analysis revealed no abnormalities in any patient.

Mean parathormone concentrations were 2.89± 1.11 pmol/L (norm 1.6–6.9 pmol/L) and revealed no signs of hyperparathyreoidism. The 25-hydroxy-vitamin D(3) serum levels were within the normal range (24.3±8.8 ng/ml; norm 9.2–45.2 ng/ml). Mean 1,25-dihydroxy-vitamin D(3) serum levels were 50.4±17.7 ng/L (norm 17–53 ng/L) and were increased in 24/64 patients (median: 69.6 ng/L, range: 56–113 ng/L), 21 of them on synthetic AA substitution (which contained 0.13–0.2 μg vitamin D3/gram protein). However, there was no correlation between nutritional supply with D3 and either 25-hydroxy-vitamin D(3) or 1,25-dihydroxy-vitamin D(3) levels. Vitamin D deficiency was not diagnosed in any of the patients. There was no correlation between vitamin D3 intake and hypercalciuria.

PAH genotype

34/57 patients carried two null mutations (genotype group 1), 23/57 patients carried at least one putative milder *PAH* mutation (genotype group 2). No significant differences between both groups were found for CD, LTD, GFR, eGFR, and proteinuria (Table 3).

Discussion

Dietary protein is a well known modulator of kidney function (Brenner et al 1982; King and Levey 1993). The effect of the PKU diet, which is characterized by a relative high protein content with a high proportion of synthetic AA, on renal function has not been previously examined. We show that adolescent and adult PKU patients may develop CKD (impaired renal function, proteinuria) and arterial hypertension. In contrast, CKD in the general population is mainly prevalent at older ages (Zhang and Rothenbacher 2008).

The RDA for the daily protein intake has changed within the last decades, and a lower nutritional protein intake is currently recommended (D-A-CH Empfehlung 2000; DGE Empfehlung 1985; DGE Empfehlung 1991). Although median total protein intake in PKU patients exceeded these RDA, the amount of total protein intake was still within the range of a typical Western diet and, thus, may not account for the development of CKD in our patients (Fouque and Aparicio 2007; Halbesma et al 2009). However, we could demonstrate that GFR decreased significantly with increasing total protein and increasing AA intake, both related to CD as well to LDT. Overall, we found hyperfiltration in only 7 % of the patients, but a decrease of GFR in 19 % of the patients. Although Phe might interfere with renal clearance of hippurate due to the competition for renal anion transporters (Enomoto and Niwa 2007), there were no correlations with plasma or urine Phe values and ERPF measured by ^{123}J-Hippuran.

Importantly, protein composition in PKU diet differs from that of healthy population and mainly derives from the synthetic AA formula. Ingestion of AA formula results in plasma peak AA concentrations (Mönch et al 1996; Gropper et al 1993), and high plasma AA concentrations have been shown to be nephrotoxic in animals, resulting in a significant decrease of GFR, an increase in albuminuria and histological changes consistent with tubular damage (Zager et al 1983). A similar pathomechanism may account for the renal damage in PKU patients.

An increase in renal protein excretion was detected in more than 30 % of the PKU patients, and microalbuminuria in 7 % of the patients. Multivariant linear regression analysis revealed a significant association of GFR measured by ^{51}Cr-EDTA with both, current total protein intake and proteinuria, indicating that protein intake and proteinuria are involved independently in the pathomechanism of renal injury in phenylketonuric patients.

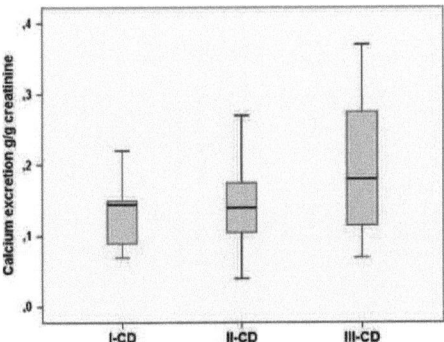

Fig. 5 Calcium excretion related to current synthetic protein intake calcium excretion was measured in 66 patients. Median urinary calcium concentration was 0.15 g/g creatinine in the group with the lowest AA intake (I-CD), 0.12 g/g creatinine in the group with the medium AA intake (II-CD), and 0.21 g/g in the group with the highest AA intake (III-CD). The correlation of calcium excretion and current synthetic protein intake (AA intake) was significant (*p*=0.008)

Table 3 Protein intake and renal function in PKU patients related to their genotype

Genotype group	Number of patients	Frequency of PAH mutations		Total protein intake (g/kg/day)	Natural protein intake (g/kg/day)	Synthetic protein intake (g/kg/day)	LDT	GFR (ml/min/1.73 m^2)	eGFR (ml/min/1.73 m^2)	Urinary protein excretion (mg/24 h)
Genotype group 1	34	p.R408W	50 %	0.98±0.25	0.27±0.18	0.72±0.35	18.0±5.1	105.4±17.5	110.0±18.8	149±299
		IVS12-1G >A	16 %							
		IVS10-11G >A	15 %							
		p.R243X	4 %							
		p.G272X	3 %							
		p.F299C	3 %							
		others	15 %							
Genotype group 2	23	p.R408W	17 %	0.96±0.24	0.30±0.18	0.66±0.34	15.4±5.6	104.7±12.4	113.0±17.4	62±74
		p.R261Q	13 %							
		p.Y414C	9 %							
		p.R413P	4 %							
		IVS10-11G >A	4 %							
		p.G272X	4 %							
		p.P281L	4 %							
		p.A395P	4 %							
		others	39 %							

Genotype group 1: patients with two null mutations, corresponding to a complete loss of residual PAH activity
Genotype group 2: patients with at least one putative milder mutation, corresponding to a certain residual PAH activity
Data are given in mean ± SD. Differences between genotype group 1 and genotype group 2 are not significant

Arterial hypertension was found in one fourth of the PKU patients, reflecting an important secondary health problem in PKU patients. Furthermore, 40 % of the patients revealed a nocturnal non-dipping status, which is known to be associated with CKD (Kastarinen et al 2010). Arterial BP was significantly associated with BMI, but not with actual or lifelong protein intake, GFR or proteinuria. More than one third of the examined patients revealed an increase in BMI. It has been reported before that obesity is a common problem in PKU patients (MacDonald et al 2011). Though, it is our experience and that of others that caloric intake in PKU patients is within normal limits (Acosta 1996). An increase in BMI in PKU patients may be due to inadequate energy expenditure (Acosta et al 2003; White et al 1982). Furthermore, our data reveal that BMI is inversely correlated with the actual total and synthetic protein intake. Obesity is a known risk factor for glomerulosclerosis (Kambham et al 2001), which is reflected by our data, revealing an association of BMI and GFR. Though, BMI was not associated proteinuria in our study. Hence, obesity is a further risk factor for CKD in PKU patients.

Calcium excretion significantly increased with increasing protein intake, mainly with increasing synthetic AA intake, whereas the time of the lifelong diet (LDT) seemed not to influence calcium excretion. A high protein intake is associated with an increase in calcium excretion (Itoh et al 1998). An increase in calcium excretion (found in 23 % of patients) could imply an additional long-term risk for PKU patients on the current diet. However nephrocalcinosis was rarely observed and the presence of hypercalciuria was not associated with diminished GFR, proteinuria or hypertension. 1,25-dihydroxy-vitamin D(3) serum concentrations were increased in 38 % of the PKU patients, but there was no correlation between the nutritional vitamin D3 supply with either 25-hydroxy-vitamin D(3) or 1,25-dihydroxy-vitamin D(3) levels. However, 1,25-dihydroxy-vitamin D(3) levels are tightly regulated on the level of synthesis, independent of nutritional supply (Anderson et al 2004). Furthermore, an increase in vitamin D(3) serum concentrations was not associated with hypercalciuria. Although actual recommendations indicate a higher vitamin D intake in adolescents and adults (German Nutrition Society 2012), none of our patients had vitamin D deficiency.

Several putative pathomechanism could explain the association of (synthetic) protein intake and a decrease in renal function. First, Phe excretion was significantly correlated with GFR and proteinuria. Although a nephrotoxic effect of Phe has not been described yet, renal damage by high urinary Phe concentrations may contribute to the development of CKD in PKU. Second, increased oxidative stress has been demonstrated in PKU patients and attributed to an increased free radical generation, a deprivation of micronutrients or an increase of phenylalanine and its metabolites (Sirtori et al 2005; Sitta et al 2009; Ribas et al 2011). Therefore, oxidative stress could be involved in the pathophysiology of the tissue damage and chronic renal injury found in PKU. Third, it has been postulated that human kidney PAH may play a significant role in phenylalanine homeostasis. PAH has been shown to be expressed in human kidneys (Lichter-Konecki et al 1999), and impaired phenylalanine hydroxylation has been observed in renal failure (Zhao et al 2012). Thus, renal PAH expression could influence renal function in PKU patients, although in our study an association with the *PAH* genotype could not be found. In contrast, hyperfiltration, a well-known mediator of renal injury associated with a high protein intake (Bernstein et al 2007; Brenner et al 1996), was not observed in our patient's cohort.

CKD in patients with PKU may benefit from an early start of treatment. Although the effects of a low-protein diet on the progression of CKD has been the subject of controversy, a protein restriction of 0.6–0.8 g/kg/day is recommended in adult patients with end-stage CKD (Fouque and Aparicio 2007). In contrast, a protein-restricted diet seems to have no significant impact on the progression of CKD in children (Wingen et al 1997; Chaturvedi and Jones 2007). Thus, at the current state of knowledge, recommendations for protein intake in PKU patients with CKD are difficult to establish. However, given the potential nephrotoxicity of AA, we recommended substitution of the AA formula in at least three daily doses (Mönch et al 1996). In addition to dietary protein restriction, ACE inhibitors or angiotensin-receptor blockers were shown to have a beneficial effect on progression of CKD (Kriz 2004). Therapy with these drugs could be beneficial in view of the high incidence of arterial hypertension in patients with PKU; however, efficacy of such treatment remains to be established in this patient population.

Conclusions

In conclusion, we found a high prevalence of proteinuria, decreased GFR, hypercalciuria, and arterial hypertension in adolescent and adult PKU patients. An increased intake of protein with a high content of synthetic AA due to lifelong prescription of a PKU diet and the presence of proteinuria were independently associated with the decrease in GFR. Although GFR was within the normal range in the whole group of patients, there was a continuous and graded relationship of both, CD and LTD, with decreasing GFR. The intake of high amounts of synthetic AA, increased oxidative stress, and local damage through high Phe excretion may contribute to renal damage in PKU. Arterial hypertension was mainly explained by increased BMI and unrelated to protein intake or proteinuria. Altogether, PKU patients constitute a high risk group for the development of CKD.

Acknowledgement We thank all patients and their parents for the participation and for their cooperation. We are grateful to Christine Gebauer and Gudrun Heide who calculated dietary protocols and dietary protein intake of all patients included in the study.

Conflict of interest None.

References

Acosta PB (1996) Recommendations for protein and energy intakes by patients with phenylketonuria. Eur J Pediatr 155(Suppl 1):S121–S124

Acosta PB, Yannicelli S, Marriage B et al (1998) Nutrient intake and growth of infants with phenylketonuria undergoing therapy. J Pediatr Gastroenterol Nutr 27:287–291

Acosta PB, Yanicelli S, Singh R et al (2003) Nutrient intakes and physical growth of children with phenylketonuria undergoing nutrition therapy. J Am Diet Assoc 103:1167–1173

Anderson PH, O'Loughlin PD, May BK, Morris HA (2004) Determinants of circulating 1,25-dihydroxyvitamin D3 levels: the role of renal synthesis and catabolism of vitamin D. J Steroid Biochem Mol Biol 89–90:111–113

Arnold GL, Vladutiu CJ, Kirby RS, Blakely EM, Deluca JM (2002) Protein insufficiency and linear growth restriction in phenylketonuria. J Pediatr 141:243–246

Bernstein AM, Treyzon L, Li Z (2007) Are high-protein, vegetable based diets safe for kidney function? A review of the literature. J Am Diet Assoc 107:644–650

Blecker S, Matsushita K, Köttgen A et al (2011) High-normal albuminuria and risk of heart failure in the community. Am J Kidney Dis 58:47–55

Brenner BM, Meyer TW, Hostetter TH (1982) Dietary protein intake and the progressive nature of kidney disease. N Engl J Med 307:652–659

Brenner BM, Lawler EV, Mackenzie HS (1996) The hyperfiltration theory: a paradigm shift in nephrology. Kidney Int 49:1774–1777

Burgard P, Bremer HJ, Bührdel P et al (1999) Rationale for the German recommendations for phenylalanine level control in phenylketonuria 1997. Eur J Pediatr 158:46–54

Chaturvedi S, Jones C (2007) Protein restriction for children with chronic renal failure. Cochrane Database Syst Rev 17(4): CD006863

DGE Empfehlung: Deutsche Gesellschaft für Ernährung (1985) *Empfehlungen für die Nährstoffzufuhr:* Umschau Verlag

DGE Empfehlung: Deutsche Gesellschaft für Ernährung (1991) *Empfehlungen für die* Nährstoffzufuhr: Umschau/Braus

D-A-CH Empfehlung: Deutsche Gesellschaft für Ernährung, Österreichische Gesellschaft für Ernährung, Schweizerische Gesellschaft für Ernährungsforschung, Schweizerische Vereinigung für Ernährung (2000) *Referenzwerte für die Nährstoffzufuhr:* Umschau/Braus

Enomoto A, Niwa T (2007) Roles of organic anion transporters in the progression of chronic renal failure. Ther Apher Dial 11(Suppl 1): S27–S31

Fouque D, Aparicio M (2007) Eleven reasons to control the protein intake of patients with chronic kidney disease. Nat Clin Pract Nephrol 3:383–392

German Nutrition Society (2012) New reference values for vitamin D. Ann Nutr Metab 60:241–246

Gropper SS, Gropper DM, Acosta PB (1993) Plasma amino acid response to ingestion of L-amino acids and whole protein. J Pediatr Gastroenterol Nutr 16:143–150

Guldberg P, Rey F, Zschocke J et al (1998) A European multicenter study of phenylalanine hydroxylase deficiency: classification of 105 mutations and a general system for genotype-based prediction of metabolic phenotype. Am J Hum Genet 63:71–79

Güttler F, Guldberg KF (1994) Mutations in the phenylalanine hydroxylase gene: genetic determinants for the phenotypic variability of hyperphenylalaninemia. Acta Paediatr 407(Suppl):46–56

Guy M, Borzomato JK, Newall RG, Kalra PA, Price CP (2009) Protein and albumin-to-creatinine ratios in random urines accurately predict 24 h protein and albumin loss in patients with kidney disease. Ann Clin Biochem 46:468–476

Halbesma N, Bakker SJ, Jansen DF et al (2009) High protein intake associates with cardiovascular events but not with loss of renal function. J Am Soc Nephrol 20:1797–1804

Hennermann JB, Vetter B, Wolf C et al (2000) Phenylketonuria and hyperphenylalaninemia in Eastern Germany: a characteristic molecular profile and 15 novel mutations. Hum Mut 15:254–260

Hoeksma M, Van Rijn M, Verkerk PH et al (2005) The intake of total protein, natural protein and protein substitute and growth of height and head circumference in Dutch infants with phenylketonuria. J Inherit Metab Dis 28:845–854

Hüseman D, Gellermann J, Vollmer I et al (1999) Long-term prognosis of hemolytic uremic syndrome and effective renal plasma flow. Pediatr Nephrol 13:672–677

Itoh R, Nishiyama N, Suyama Y (1998) Dietary protein intake and urinary excretion of calcium: a cross-sectional study in a healthy Japanese population. Am J Clin Nutr 67:438–444

Jia Y, Hwang SY, House JD, Ogborn MR, Weiler HA, Karmin O, Aukema HM (2010) Long-term high intake of whole proteins results in renal damage in pigs. J Nutr 140: 1646–1652

Kambham N, Markowitz GS, Valeri AM (2001) Obesity-related glomerulopathy: an emerging epidemic. Kidney Int 59:1498–1509

Kastarinen H, Vasunta RL, Ukkola O, Kesäniemi YA (2010) Glomerular filtration rate is related to dipping pattern in ambulatory blood pressure monitoring—a cross-sectional population-based study. J Hum Hypertens 24:247–253

King AJ, Levey AS (1993) Dietary protein and renal function. J Am Soc Nephrol 3:1723–1737

Kooman JP (2009) Estimation of renal function in patients with chronic kidney disease. J Magn Reson Imaging 30:1341–1346

Krauch G, Müller E, Anninos A, Bremer HJ (1996) Comparison of the protein quality of dietetically treated phenylketonuria patients with the recommendations of the WHO expert consultation. Eur J Pediatr 155(Suppl 1):S153–S157

Kriz W (2004) Podocytes as a target for treatment with ACE inhibitors and/or angiotensin-receptor blockers. Kidney Int 65:333–334

Lichter-Konecki U, Hipke CM, Konecki DS (1999) Human phenylalanine hydroxylase gene expression in kidney and other nonhepatic tissues. Mol Genet Metab 67:308–316

MacDonald A, Rocha JC, van Rijn M, Feillet F (2011) Nutrition in phenylketonuria. Mol Genet Metab 104(Suppl):S10–S18

Manz F, Schmidt H, Schärer K, Bickel H (1977) Acid-base status in dietary treatment of phenylketonuria. Pediatr Res 11:1084–1087

Mönch E, Herrmann ME, Brösicke H, Schöffer A, Keller M (1996) Utilisation of amino acid mixtures in adolescents with phenylketonuria. Eur J Pediatr 155(Suppl 1):S115–S120

O'Brien E, Asmar R, Beilin L et al (2005) Practice guidelines of the European Society of Hypertension for clinic, ambulatory and self blood pressure measurement. J Hypertens 23:697–701

Parati G, Pickering TG (2009) Home blood-pressure monitoring: US and European consensus. Lancet 373:876–878

Ribas GS, Sitta A, Wajner M, Vargas CR (2011) Oxidative stress in phenylketonuria: what is the evidence? Cell Mol Neurobiol 31:653–662

Schena FP (2011) Management of patients with chronic kidney disease. Intern Emerg Med 6(Suppl 1):77–83

Schwartz GJ, Muñoz A, Schneider MF et al (2009) New equations to estimate GFR in children with CKAD. J Am Soc Nephrol 20:629–637

Scriver CR, Kaufman S (2001) Phenylalanine hydroxylase deficiency. In Scriver CR, Beaudet AL, Sly W, Valle D, Childs B, Vogelstein B (eds). The metabolic and molecular basis of inherited disease. McGraw-Hill, 1667–1724

Sirtori LR, Dutra-Filho CS, Fitarelli D et al (2005) Oxidative stress in patients with phenylketonuria. Biochim Biophys Acta 1740:68–73

Sitta A, Barschak AG, Deon M et al (2009) L-Carnitine blood levels and oxidative stress in treated phenylketonuric patients. Cell Mol Neurobiol 29:211–218

Staples A, LeBlond R, Watkins S, Wong C, Brandt J (2010) Validation of the revised Schwartz estimating equation in a predominantly non-CKD population. Pediatr Nephrol 25:2321–2326

White JE, Kronmal RA, Acosta PB (1982) Excess weight among children with phenylketonuria. J Am Coll Nutr 1:293–303

Wingen AM, Fabian-Bach C, Mehls O (1997) Randomised multicentre study of a low-protein diet on the progression of chronic renal failure in children. European study group of nutritional treatment of chronic renal failure in childhood. Lancet 349:1117–1123

Wühl E, Witte K, Soergel M, Mehls O, Schaefer F (2002) German working group on pediatric hypertension: distribution of 24-h ambulatory blood pressure in children: normalized reference values and role of body dimensions. J Hypertens 20:1995–2007

Zager RA, Johannes G, Tuttle SE, Sharma HM (1983) Acute amino acid nephrotoxicity. J Lab Clin Med 101:130–140

Zhang QL, Rothenbacher D (2008) Prevalence of chronic kidney disease in population-based studies: systematic review. BMC Publ Health 8:117

Zhao YY, Liu J, Cheng XL, Bai X, Lin RC (2012) Urinary metabonomics study on biochemical changes in an experimental model of chronic renal failure by adenine based on UPLC Q-TOF/MS. Clin Chim Acta 413:642–649

2.3. PUBLIKATION 3: **Hennermann JB**, Bührer C, Blau N, Vetter B, Mönch E. Long-term treatment with tetrahydrobiopterin increases phenylalanine tolerance in children with severe phenotype of phenylketonuria. 2005. Mol Genet Metab 86:S86-S90. DOI 10.1016/j.ymgme.2005.05.013

Reprinted from: Molecular Genetics and Metabolism 2005, Volume 86 Suppl 1, page S86-90, with permission from Elsevier Inc., 2005, provided by Copyright Clearance Center

BH4 stellt eine neue Option in der Behandlung der PKU dar. Nach der Erstbeschreibung der BH4-responsiven PKU in 1999 (Kure et al. 1999) wurden zunächst ausschließlich Patienten mit einer milden PKU beschrieben, die auf BH4 ansprachen. In dieser Studie untersuchten wir erstmals das Langzeit-Ansprechen auf BH4 bei Patienten mit einem schweren PKU-Phänotyp.

Wir führten einen BH4-Belastungstest bei 40 im Neugeborenenscreening diagnostizierten Neugeborenen mit einer Phe-Serumkonzentration >240 µmol/L durch. 18 der 40 Patienten zeigten ein Ansprechen im BH4-Belastungstest. 5 dieser 18 BH4-responsiven Patienten wiesen einen schweren PKU-Phänotyp auf, entsprechend einer Phe-Toleranz von <20 mg/kg KG/Tag und einer Phe-Serumkonzentration von >1000 µmol/L bei Diagnosestellung. Diese 5 Patienten wurden über einen Zeitraum von 24 Monaten (5,5-29 Monate) mit BH4 in einer Dosierung von 20 mg/kg KG/Tag behandelt. Alter bei Behandlungsbeginn war im Median 1,2 Monate. Alle 5 Patienten zeigten ein dauerhaftes Ansprechen auf BH4: bei stabiler Stoffwechseleinstellung konnte die Phe-Toleranz unter der BH4-Therapie deutlich gesteigert werden. Vor Beginn der BH4-Therapie betrug die tägliche Phe-Toleranz 18-19 mg/kg, sie stieg unter BH4-Gabe auf 30-80 mg/kg an und fiel nach Beendigung der BH4-Therapie wieder auf 12-17 mg/kg ab. Die Mutationsanalysen ergaben eine Compound-Heterozygosität für eine Nullmutation und eine variante *PAH-M*utation bei vier Patienten sowie eine Homozygosität für eine variante *PAH-M*utation bei einem Patienten.

Mit diesen Daten konnten wir erstmals nachweisen, dass eine BH4-Responsivität nicht auf milde PKU-Phänotypen beschränkt ist, sondern dass auch Patienten mit einem schweren PKU-Phänotyp BH4-responsiv sein können und auf eine Langzeitbehandlung mit BH4 ansprechen.

Long-term treatment with tetrahydrobiopterin increases phenylalanine tolerance in children with severe phenotype of phenylketonuria

Julia B. Hennermann [a,*], Christoph Bührer [a,b], Nenad Blau [c], Barbara Vetter [a], Eberhard Mönch [a]

[a] *Otto Heubner Center for Pediatric and Adolescent Medicine, Charité University Medical Center, Campus Virchow-Klinikum, Berlin, Germany*
[b] *University Children's Hospital, Basel, Switzerland*
[c] *Division of Clinical Chemistry and Biochemistry, University Children's Hospital, Zürich, Switzerland*

Received 30 April 2005; received in revised form 25 May 2005; accepted 26 May 2005
Available online 26 July 2005

Abstract

Hyperphenylalaninemia caused by phenylalanine hydroxylase (PAH) deficiency requires lifelong rigorous diet starting in early infancy to prevent severe neurodevelopmental handicap. In a considerable number of children with mild hyperphenylalaninemia, long-term tetrahydrobiopterin (BH4) treatment significantly improves phenylalanine (phe) tolerance, but it has never been investigated in classic phenylketonuria (PKU). We performed a BH4-loading test in 40 consecutive infants with phe serum concentrations exceeding 240 µM, who had been detected by newborn screening programs. Eighteen out of 40 infants were found to be BH4 responsive. Five of them, responding to the neonatal BH4-loading test, showed a phe tolerance of less than 20 mg/kg/day and a phe pretreatment level of >1000 µM. They were treated with BH4 (20 mg/kg/day) over a period of 24 months. All five children had a sustained response to BH4, allowing substantial easing of dietary restrictions. Before BH4 treatment daily phe tolerance was 18–19 mg/kg, increasing to 30–80 mg/kg on BH4 treatment and decreasing again to 12–17 mg/kg after termination of BH4 treatment. Mutation analysis revealed compound heterozygosity for a putative null and a variant *PAH* mutation in four patients and homozygosity for a variant *PAH* mutation in one patient. We conclude that BH4 sensitivitiy is not restricted to mild hyperphenylalaninemia and that long-term BH4 treatment may also improve phenylalanine tolerance in a considerable number of children with a more severe PKU phenotype.
© 2005 Elsevier Inc. All rights reserved.

Keywords: Tetrahydrobiopterin; BH4; BH4-responsive; Hyperphenylalaninemia; Phenylketonuria; Classic; PKU

Introduction

Hyperphenylalaninemia is caused either by phenylalanine hydroxylase (PAH)[1] deficiency (Online Mendelian Inheritance in Man number 261600) or by a defect in the synthesis or regeneration of its coenzyme tetrahydrobiopterin (BH4). While the latter requires supplementation of BH4 and various BH4-dependent synthesized neurotransmitters, normal psychomotor development can be achieved in PAH deficiency by early institution of phenylalanine (phe)-restricted diet. In 1999, Kure et al. reported for the first time on four infants with a novel subtype of BH4-responsive hyperphenylalaninemia. These infants showed a decrease of phe concentrations after oral administration of BH4 but displayed a normal BH4 metabolism and compound heterozygosity for

---

* Corresponding author. Fax: +49 30 450566918.
E-mail address: julia.hennermann@charite.de (J.B. Hennermann).
[1] *Abbreviations used:* BH4, tetrahydrobiopterin; bw, body weight; MHPA, mild hyperphenylalaninemia; phe, phenylalanine; PAH, phenylalanine hydroxylase; PKU, phenylketonuria.

1096-7192/$ - see front matter © 2005 Elsevier Inc. All rights reserved.
doi:10.1016/j.ymgme.2005.05.013

different *PAH* mutations [1]. Since then, several infants with BH4-responsive PAH deficiency have been reported [2–9]. Different mechanisms had been discussed to cause BH4-responsive PAH deficiency [2]. All hypotheses put forward to date assume an association with specific, mainly milder *PAH* mutations. Of the almost 500 *PAH* mutations known, more than 35 have been associated with BH4 responsiveness [3–5,10,11].

Muntau et al. [4] showed that BH4 significantly lowered serum phe concentrations in the majority of patients with mild hyperphenylalaninemia (MHPA), while no patients with classic phenylketonuria (PKU) had a response. This is in line with previous reports, none of which found BH4 responsiveness in patients with classic PKU [1,6–8]. BH4 responsiveness in infants with classic PKU has been reported only twice, for the first time by our group [12] and recently by Matalon et al. [13]. Long-term BH4 treatment has been described several times in children with MHPA [6,8,14,15], but was never proved in children with classic PKU. We now report for the first time the effect of long-term BH4 treatment in children with a severe PKU phenotype.

Methods and patients

BH4 loading test

Over a period of 5 years, between October 1999 and October 2004, we performed the BH4 loading test in all consecutive infants with phe serum concentrations exceeding 240 µmol/L, as detected by newborn screening programs ($n=40$). BH4 test was performed at the median age of 11 days of life. All infants received the fully active (6R)-BH4 (Schircks Laboratories, Jona, Switzerland; chemical purity 99.5%, application form: tablets solved in fluids) by mouth in one dose of 20 mg/kg body weight (bw) after a fasting period of 4 h. Phe serum concentrations were measured before, 4, 8, and in 32/40 children, 24 h after the application of BH4. During the BH4 test infants were still regularly breast- or bottle-fed. BH4 responsiveness was defined as a drop of serum phe levels 8–24 h after BH4 application by more than 30% from the value obtained before the administration of BH4 [4,9]. A defect of BH4 synthesis or regeneration was excluded in all 40 infants by measuring dihydropteridine reductase activity in dried blood filter card samples and by determination of pterins in urine samples collected before and during BH4 loading tests.

Classification

Adapted to previously established criteria, hyperphenylalaninemia was classified by using pretreatment phe levels [>1200 µM = classic PKU; 900–1200 µM = mild PKU; <900 µM = MHPA] and maximum daily phe tolerance [<20 mg/kg = classic PKU; 20–25 mg/kg = mild PKU; >25 mg/kg = MHPA] [16,17]. Pretreatment phe levels were established at a median age of 9.5 days (4–12 days of life) before starting any diet or medication. Classic PKU was diagnosed in 23 children, mild PKU in five children, and MHPA in 12 children. Two children (IDs 1 and 2) with the clinical phenotype of classic PKU but a milder genotype carrying the variant mutation Y414C were classified as "atypical" classic PKU. Two children (IDs 4 and 5) showed phe pretreatment levels between 1000 and 1200 µM and a low phe tolerance of <20 mg/kg/day. Due to their genotype they were classified as mild PKU, but—as their clinical course resembled that of children with classic PKU—they were included into the study (Tables 1 and 2).

Laboratory methods

Serum amino acids were analyzed by automated cation exchange chromatography (Biotronic/Eppendorf). Pterins in urine were analyzed by HPLC [18] and dihydropteridine reductase activity was measured in whole blood in filter cards as described previously [19]. Genomic DNA was amplified by polymerase chain reaction and sequenced as described previously [20]. Parental DNA analysis was performed to exclude monoallelic double heterozygosity.

Long-term BH4 treatment

Long-term BH4 treatment was started in all BH4-responsive PKU children with initial phe levels >1000 µM and a phe tolerance of less than 20 mg/kg (IDs 1–5). As there was no need for strong phe-restricted diet, the remaining children with mild PKU or MHPA (IDs 6–18) did not receive BH4 treatment. Long-term BH4 treatment was started at a median age of 9.25 months (from 2 weeks to 42 months) and continued over a median time of 24 months (5.5–29 months). BH4 was given in a dose of 10 mg/kg bw twice a day. Phe and tyrosine serum concentrations were measured weekly or fortnightly. Phe tolerance was evaluated by repeated 3 day dietary protocols. Side effects and positive effects of BH4 treatment were controlled regularly by interviews.

Results

The BH4 loading test revealed a significant decline of plasma phe concentrations in 18/40 infants with hyperphenylalaninemia: in 3/23 infants with classic/atypical classic PKU, in 4/5 infants with mild PKU, and in 11/12 infants with MHPA (Table 1). In all BH4-responsive children, a median decrease of phe serum concentrations of 46% (12.3–82.6%) was achieved 8 h after BH4 application, and of 46% (31.6–59.6%) 24 h after BH4

Table 1
Children with BH4-responsive PKU, as detected by newborn screening

ID	PKU-form	Genotype	
		Allele 1	Allele 2
1	Atypical classic PKU	Y414C[a,b]	R252W[c]
2	Atypical classic PKU	Y414C[a,b]	R408W[c]
3	Classic PKU	**A309V**[d]	R408W[c]
4	Mild PKU[e]	R261Q[a,b]	R261Q[a,b]
5	Mild PKU[e]	**D129G**[f]	R408W[c]
6	Mild PKU	I306V[b,f]	?
7	Mild PKU	?	R408W[c]
8	MHPA	A403V[b,f]	R408W[c]
9	MHPA	A403V[b,f]	L41F[d]
10	MHPA	**P211T**[d]	**P211T**[d]
11	MHPA	A403V[b,f]	IVS10nt-11g>a[c]
12	MHPA	E390G[b,f]	E390G[b,f]
13	MHPA	A403V[b,f]	K274fsdel11bp[c]
14	MHPA	**S110L**[d]	P281L[c]
15	MHPA	A403V[b,f]	R408W[c]
16	MHPA	?	R408W[c]
17	MHPA	A403V[b,f]	A300S[b,f]
18	MHPA	nd	nd

nd, not determined.
Mutations are printed in bold: newly identified mutations in BH4-sensitive PKU.
[a] Variant mutation [10,17].
[b] Previously described in BH4-responsive PAH deficiency [3].
[c] Putative null mutation [10,17].
[d] Unclassified mutation [10,17].
[e] Phe pretreatment levels were >1000 μM, but phe tolerance was <20 mg/kg/day.
[f] Mild mutation [10,17].

Table 2
Maximum phe pretreatment level and decrease of phe levels during initial phe loading test in children with BH4-responsive PKU and low phe tolerance (<20 mg/kg)

ID	Maximum pretreatment phe concentration (μmol/L)	Effect of BH4 on phe decrease (%)		Sex
		8 h	24 h	
1	1816	46.2	na	Female
2	1459	34.2	na	Male
3	1316	25.4	43.8	Female
4	1150	22.1	58.4	Male
5	1077	82.2	na	Male

na, not applicable.

application. Tyrosine concentrations remained unchanged in all children. Mutation analysis revealed heterozygosity for *PAH* mutations in 11 children and homozygosity in three children with BH4 responsiveness. In three of the children only one *PAH* mutation was identified, although all exons and splice sites had been sequenced. S110L, D129G, P211T, and A309V were newly identified in our patients to be BH4-responsive missense mutations (Table 1).

Long-term BH4 treatment was performed in 5/18 children with BH4-responsive PAH deficiency and a low phe tolerance of <20 mg/kg (Tables 2 and 3). All five children had a sustained response to long-term BH4

Table 3
Course of long-term BH4 therapy in BH4-responsive children with classic and mild PKU

ID	Phe tolerance (mg/kg/day)		Phe tolerance (mg/day)			Median phe concentrations (μmol/L)			Age at start of BH4 therapy (months)	Duration of BH4 therapy (months)
	Before (without) BH4 therapy	On BH4 therapy	After (without) BH4 therapy	Before (without) BH4 therapy	On BH4 therapy	After (without) BH4 therapy	Before (without) BH4 therapy	On BH4 therapy	After (without) BH4 therapy	
1	19	35	16	220	420	260	143 (18–557) n = 65	299 (61–1065)[a] n = 78	309 (157–587)[a] n = 21	18	24
2	19	80	12	100	850	200	77 (30–157)[b] n = 6	314 (36–726) n = 52	335 (67–757) n = 28	1.2	29
3	–[c]	40	17	–[c]	240	190	–[c]	293 (30–720) n = 49	327 (18–684) n = 42	0.5	8
4	–[c]	30	17	–[c]	240	190	–[c]	190 (30–490) n = 21	246 (61–636) n = 59	0.5	5.5
5	18	120	20	180	1800	340	208 (18–775) n = 75	249 (54–799)[a] n = 51	340 (182–502) n = 39	42	24

[a] The slight increase of median phe serum concentrations on long-term BH4 treatment is associated with commencement of kindergarten and subsequent recurrent febrile infections.
[b] BH4 treatment was started already at the age of 1.2 months. Therefore only few data on phe levels before BH4 treatment do occur and they cannot be compared to those on BH4 treatment.
[c] In patients 3 and 4, BH4 treatment was started already at the age of 2 weeks. Therefore data on treatment before BH4-treatment do not exist.

treatment, allowing substantial easing of dietary restrictions. Before BH4 treatment daily median phe tolerance was 18 mg/kg, increasing to 40 mg/kg on BH4 treatment and decreasing again to 17 mg/kg after termination of BH4 treatment (Table 3). Serum phe concentrations increased immediately in children who had not received BH4 or had vomited it. Serum phe concentrations also increased in catabolic situations, such as fever or enteritis. As in children managed by diet alone, median phe serum concentrations increased slightly in all children with age, associated with commencement of kindergarten and subsequent recurrent febrile infections, independently if they were on long-term BH4 treatment or on diet alone.

No side effects were observed during BH4 short- and long-term treatment. In one boy, parents reported of hyperactivity and sleeplessness after the first dosage of BH4. These symptoms resolved on the second day of treatment and never recurred. Growth, length, and head circumference were within the percentiles for age and sex. All children showed normal mental and motor development, documented by regular neurodevelopmental testing. All parents reported of an increase of quality of life due to the stop or relaxation of protein-restricted diet.

Discussion

This is the first report of the effectiveness of long-term BH4 treatment in children with a severe PKU phenotype. In contrast to previous reports [4,21], our data show that responsiveness to BH4 is not restricted to mild PKU but may occur in severe phenotypes as well, defined as children with a low phe tolerance of <20 mg/kg. All children showed a sustained response to long-term BH4 treatment, resulting in a distinct relaxation of phe-restricted diet and hence an improvement of the quality of life. Remarkably, none of the infants with a BH4-responsive severe PKU phenotype carried two null mutations, but in spite of the severe phenotype one variant or mild PAH mutation in trans with a null mutation. A comparable result was reported by Matalon et al. [13] showing compound heterozygosity for one mild or variant PAH mutation and one classic PAH mutation in all children with BH4-responsive classic PKU. As shown by our data and also reported by Matalon et al. [12,13], one common variant mutation in classic BH4-responsive PKU is Y414C, which is associated with all different PKU phenotypes [17]. Also children with mild PKU and MHPA carried at least one mild or variant PAH mutation, with a high frequency of A403V in children with BH4-responsive MHPA. We identified four new BH4-responsive mutations: A309V in classic PKU, D129G in mild PKU, and P211T and S110L in MHPA. Except D129G, which has been associated with a milder phenotype, these newly described BH4-responsive PAH mutations are still unclassified [10,17]. Considering that P211T occurred in homozygosity and that A309V, D129G, and S110L occurred in trans with a putative BH4-non-responsive null mutation, these PAH mutations may account for BH4 responsiveness. S110L is located in the N-terminal regulatory PAH domain, while D129G, P211T, and A309V are located in the catalytic PAH domain.

The effect of BH4 has been explained by several possible mechanisms [2]. BH4-responsive mutations may be located within or near the BH4 binding regions [22], but none of our newly identified BH4-responsive mutations are located within that region. Moreover, mutations in the catalytic domain of PAH may alter the tertiary structure of PAH, resulting in a K_m-variant of PAH which is activated by BH4 by stabilizing the PAH tetramer [6,7]. But as only a few of our newly identified BH4-responsive mutations are located within the catalytic PAH domain, further mechanisms may account for the BH4 responsiveness. Kure et al. [23] recently indicated that in vivo suboptimal physiological BH4 concentrations may occur and that wild-type and mutant residual PAH activity may be enhanced by BH4 supplementation. This mechanism may explain the effect of BH4 in children with a severe PKU phenotype. Although all children with a severe PKU phenotype and BH4 responsiveness carried at least one milder or variant PAH mutation, the severe PKU phenotype was evident in these patients. We speculate that an inconsistent expression of two different PAH alleles with a dominance of the null mutation may result in a severe PKU phenotype. After the application of BH4 the dominant-negative effect may be compensated resulting in a decrease of phe levels. As null mutations may not be stimulated by BH4 [5], BH4 responsiveness may only occur in those children with a severe PKU phenotype who carry at least one mild or variant mutation.

Presenting the data on the long-term BH4 treatment in patients with a severe PKU phenotype, we conclude that BH4 responsiveness is not only restricted to mild PKU and may improve phenylalanine tolerance in children with a severe PKU phenotype as well. These data have implications for clinical classification schemes and therapeutic issues. However, on BH4 treatment children significantly could ease their phe-restricted diet. The increased phe tolerance by BH4 eases management and improves the quality of life. Therefore, BH4 responsiveness should be considered in all infants with elevated phe, regardless of baseline concentrations and phe tolerance. Long-term BH4 treatment may be considered in all children with a positive BH4 loading test in infancy regardless of baseline phe tolerance and at least one milder or variant PAH mutation.

Acknowledgments

We thank all the children and their parents for participating in the study and for their cooperation. The work of the dieticians C. Gebauer and G. Heide is gratefully acknowledged. This work was supported in part by the Swiss National Science Foundation Grant No. 310000-107500 (to N.B.).

References

[1] S. Kure, D.-C. Hou, T. Ohura, H. Iwamoto, S. Suzuki, N. Sugiyama, N. Sugiyama, O. Sakamoto, K. Fujii, Y. Matsubara, K. Narisawa, Tetrahydrobiopterin-responsive phenylalanine hydroxylase deficiency, J. Pediatr. 135 (1999) 375–378.
[2] N. Blau, H. Erlandsen, The metabolic and molecular bases of tetrahydrobiopterin-responsive phenylalanine hydroxylase deficiency, Mol. Genet. Metab. 82 (2004) 101–111.
[3] N. Blau. International Database of BH4-responsive HPA/PKU [<http://www.bh4.org/biopku.html>/>.
[4] A.C. Muntau, W. Röschinger, M. Habich, H. Demmelmair, B. Hoffmann, C.P. Sommerhoff, A.A. Roscher, Tetrahydrobiopterin as an alternative treatment for mild PKU, N. Engl. J. Med. 347 (2002) 2122–2132.
[5] L.J.M. Spaapen, M.E. Rubio-Gonzalbo, Tetrahydrobiopterin-responsive phenylalanine hydroxylase deficiency, state of the art, Mol. Genet. Metab. 78 (2003) 93–99.
[6] F.K. Trefz, C. Aulela-Scholz, N. Blau, Successful treatment of phenylketonuria with tetrahydrobiopterin, Eur. J. Pediatr. 160 (2001) 315.
[7] M. Lindner, D. Haas, J. Zschocke, P. Burgard, Tetrahydrobiopterin responsiveness in phenylketonuria differs between patients with the same genotype, Mol. Genet. Metab. 73 (2001) 104–106.
[8] R. Steinfeld, A. Kohlschütter, J. Zschocke, M. Lindner, K. Ullrich, Z. Lukacs, Tetrahydrobiopterin monotherapy for phenylketonuria patients with common mild mutations, Eur. J. Pediatr. 161 (2002) 403–405.
[9] C. Bernegger, N. Blau, High frequency of tetrahydrobiopterin-responsiveness among hyperphenylalaninemias: a study of 1919 patients observed from 1988 to 2002, Mol. Genet. Metab. 77 (2002) 304–313.
[10] The PAH database: <http://www.pahdb.mcgill.ca/>.
[11] Tetrahydrobiopterin home page: <http://www.bh4.org/>.
[12] J.B. Hennermann, B. Vetter, A.E. Kulozik, E. Mönch, Partial and total tetrahydrobiopterin-responsiveness in classical and mild phenlyketonuria (PKU), J. Inherit. Metab. Dis. 25 (Suppl. 1) (2002) 21.
[13] R. Matalon, R. Koch, K. Michals-Matalon, K. Moseley, S. Surendran, S. Tyring, H. Erlandsen, A. Gamez, R. Stevens, A. Romstad, L. Møller, F. Güttler, Biopterin responsive phenylalanine hydroxylase deficiency, Genet. Med. 6 (2004) 27–32.
[14] R. Cerone, M.C. Schiaffino, A.R. Fantasia, M. Perfumo, L. Birk Moller, N. Blau, Long-term follow-up of a patient with mild tetrahydrobiopterin-responsive phenylketonuria, Mol. Genet. Metab. 81 (2004) 37–139.
[15] H. Shintaku, S. Kure, T. Ohura, Y. Okano, M. Ohwada, N. Sugiyama, N. Sakura, I. Yoshida, M. Yoshino, Y. Matsubara, K. Suzuki, K. Aoki, T. Kitagawa, Long-term treatment and diagnosis of tetrahydrobiopterin-responsive phenylalanine hydroxylase gene, Pediatr. Res. 55 (2004) 425–430.
[16] F. Güttler, K.F. Guldberg, Mutations in the phenylalanine hydroxylase gene: genetic determinants for the phenotypic variability of hyperphenylalaninemia, Acta Paediatr. 407 (Suppl.) (1994) 46–56.
[17] P. Guldberg, F. Rey, J. Zschocke, V. Romano, B. François, L. Michiels, K. Ullrich, G.F. Hoffmann, P. Burgard, H. Schmidt, C. Meli, E. Riva, I. Dianzani, A. Ponzone, J. Rey, F. Güttler, A European multicenter study of phenylalanine hydroxylase deficiency: classification of 105 mutations and a general system for genotype-based prediction of metabolic phenotype, Am. J. Hum. Genet. 63 (1998) 71–79.
[18] H.C. Curtius, N. Blau, T. Kuster, Pterins, in: F.A. Hommes (Ed.), Techniques in Diagnostic Human Biochemical Genetics, Wiley-Liss, New York, 1991, pp. 377–396.
[19] N. Arai, K. Narisawa, H. Hayakawa, K. Tada, Hyperphenylalaninemia due to dihydropteridine reductase deficiency: diagnosis by enzyme assay on dried blood spots, Pediatrics 98 (1982) 426–430.
[20] J.B. Hennermann, B. Vetter, C. Wolf, E. Windt, P. Bührdel, J. Seidel, E. Mönch, A.E. Kulozik, Phenylketonuria and hyperphenylalaninemia in Eastern Germany: a characteristic molecular profile and 15 novel mutations, Hum. Mutat. 15 (2000) 254–260.
[21] M. Lindner, R. Steinfeld, P. Burgard, A. Schulze, E. Mayatepek, J. Zschocke, Tetrahydrobiopterin sensitivity in German patients with mild phenylalanine hydroxylase deficiency, Hum. Mutat. 21 (2003) 400.
[22] H. Erlandsen, R.C. Stevens, A structural hypothesis for BH4 responsiveness in patients with mild forms of hyperphenylalaninemia and phenylketonuria, J. Inherit. Metab. Dis. 24 (2001) 213–230.
[23] S. Kure, K. Sato, K. Fujii, Y. Aoki, Y. Suzuki, S. Kato, Y. Matsubara, Wild-type phenylalanine hydroxylase activity is enhanced by tetrahydrobiopterin supplementation in vivo: an implication for therapeutic basis of tetrahydrobiopterin-responsive phenylalanine hydroxylase deficiency, Mol. Genet. Metab. 83 (2004) 150–156.

2.4. PUBLIKATION 4: Trefz FK, Burton BK, Longo N, Martinez-Pardo Casanova M, Gruskin DJ, Dorenbaum A, Kakkis ED, Crombez EA, Grange DK, Harmatz P, Levy HL, Lipson MH, Milanowski A, Randolph LM, Vockley G, Whitley CB, Wolff JA, Bebchuk J, Christ-Schmidt H, **Hennermann JB**. Efficacy of sapropterin dihydrochloride in increasing phenylalanine tolerance in children with phenylketonuria: a Phase III, randomized, double-blind, placebo-controlled study. 2009. J Pediatr 154:700-707. DOI 10.1016/j.jpeds.2008.11.040

Reprinted from: The Journal of Pediatrics 2009, Volume 154 (5), page 700-7, with permission from Mosby Inc., 2009, provided by Copyright Clearance Center

Ziel dieser Studie war die Untersuchung der Wirkung von Sapropterin-Dihydrochlorid (Sapropterin), der synthetisch hergestellten Form von BH4, auf eine Steigerung der Phe-Toleranz bei Kindern mit PKU im Alter zwischen 4-18 Jahren. Diese multizentrische, internationale, randomisierte und Placebo-kontrollierte Doppelblind-Studie wurde in zwei Teilen durchgeführt. Im ersten Studienteil wurde das Ansprechen auf Sapropterin bei insgesamt 90 Patienten über einen Zeitraum von 8 Tagen untersucht. 50 von 90 Patienten zeigten ein Ansprechen auf Sapropterin mit einem Abfall der Phe-Blutwerte um 64,0 ± 17,5%. 46 dieser 50 Patienten wurden in den zweiten Teil der Studie eingeschlossen. In diesem Studienteil wurden diese 46 Patienten randomisiert (3:1) mit 20 mg/kg KG/Tag Sapropterin oder mit Placebo über einen Zeitraum von zehn Wochen behandelt. Drei Wochen nach Randomisierung wurde die Phe-Zufuhr alle zwei Wochen abhängig von den aktuellen Phe-Blutwerten mittels Gabe von Milch- oder Eiweißpulver adaptiert.

In den ersten drei Wochen nach Randomisierung zeigte sich in der Sapropterin-Gruppe ein signifikanter Abfall der Phe-Blutkonzentration von 149 ± 134 µmol/L, in der Placebo-Gruppe zeigte sich dagegen keine signifikante Veränderung der Phe-Blutkonzentration. Über einen Zeitraum von zehn Wochen konnte die Phe-Zufuhr bei den Patienten, die Sapropterin erhielten, signifikant um 20,9 ± 15,4 mg/kg KG/Tag gesteigert werden, bei den Patienten der Placebo-Gruppe zeigte sich keine signifikante Steigerung der Phe-Zufuhr. Die Differenz der Phe-Steigerung zwischen der Sapropterin- und der Placebo-Gruppe war signifikant mit 17,7 ± 4,5 mg/kg KG/Tag. 12 der 33 Patienten (36%) der Sapropterin-Gruppe tolerierten einen Anstieg der Phe-Zufuhr von ≤10 mg/kg KG/Tag, 10 Patienten (30%) einen Anstieg von 11-30 mg/kg KG/Tag und 11 Patienten (33%) einen Anstieg von 31-50 mg/kg KG/Tag. Keiner der 12 Patienten der Placebo-Gruppe tolerierte einen Anstieg der Phe-Toleranz auf ≥10 mg/kg KG/Tag, 7/12 Patienten zeigten keinen Anstieg der Phe-Toleranz. Schwere Nebenwirkungen traten nicht auf; häufigere Nebenwirkungen in der Sapropterin-Gruppe waren Kopfschmerzen, Rhinorrhoe sowie gastrointestinale Probleme.

Anhand dieser Daten konnten wir nachweisen, dass bei BH4-responsiven PKU-Patienten unter der Behandlung mit Sapropterin die individuelle Phe-Toleranz bei gleichzeitig stabilen Phe-Blutkonzentrationen signifikant gesteigert werden kann.

Efficacy of Sapropterin Dihydrochloride in Increasing Phenylalanine Tolerance in Children with Phenylketonuria: A Phase III, Randomized, Double-Blind, Placebo-Controlled Study

FRIEDRICH K. TREFZ, MD, BARBARA K. BURTON, MD, NICOLA LONGO, MD, PHD, MERCEDES MARTINEZ-PARDO CASANOVA, MD, DANIEL J. GRUSKIN, MD, ALEX DORENBAUM, MD, EMIL D. KAKKIS, MD, PHD, ERIC A. CROMBEZ, MD, DOROTHY K. GRANGE, MD, PAUL HARMATZ, MD, MARK H. LIPSON, MD, ANDRZEJ MILANOWSKI, MD, PHD, LINDA MARIE RANDOLPH, MD, JERRY VOCKLEY, MD, PHD, CHESTER B. WHITLEY, MD, PHD, JON A. WOLFF, MD, JUDITH BEBBUK, ScD, HEIDI CHRIST-SCHMIDT, MSE, AND JULIA B. HENNERMANN, MD, FOR THE SAPROPTERIN STUDY GROUP*

Objective To evaluate the ability of sapropterin dihydrochloride (pharmaceutical preparation of tetrahydrobiopterin) to increase phenylalanine (Phe) tolerance while maintaining adequate blood Phe control in 4- to 12-year-old children with phenylketonuria (PKU).
Study design This international, double-blind, randomized, placebo-controlled study screened for sapropterin response among 90 enrolled subjects in Part 1. In Part 2, 46 responsive subjects with PKU were randomized (3:1) to sapropterin, 20 mg/kg/d, or placebo for 10 weeks while continuing on a Phe-restricted diet. After 3 weeks, a dietary Phe supplement was added every 2 weeks if Phe control was adequate.
Results The mean (±SD) Phe supplement tolerated by the sapropterin group had increased significantly from the pretreatment amount (0 mg/kg/d) to 20.9 (±15.4) mg/kg/d ($P < .001$) at the last visit at which subjects had adequate blood Phe control (<360 μmol/L), up to week 10. Over the 10-week period, the placebo group tolerated only an additional 2.9 (±4.0) mg/kg/d Phe supplement; the mean difference from the sapropterin group (±SE) was 17.7 ± 4.5 mg/kg/d ($P < .001$). No severe or serious related adverse events were observed.
Conclusions Sapropterin is effective in increasing Phe tolerance while maintaining blood Phe control and has an acceptable safety profile in this population of children with PKU. *(J Pediatr 2009;154:700-7)*

P henylketonuria (PKU) is an autosomal recessive, inborn error of amino acid metabolism caused by mutations in the gene encoding phenylalanine hydroxylase (PAH).[1] More than 500 different mutations have been identified[2] that give rise to PAH deficiency and a wide range of clinical phenotypes, from mild hyperphenylalaninaemia and mild PKU to severe "classic" PKU.[1] Overall, PKU occurs in about 1 in 15 000 births, with considerable variation in incidence among different populations.[1,3]

In infants and children, impaired ability to metabolize phenylalanine (Phe) from dietary protein leads to abnormally high blood Phe levels which have a direct, damaging effect on brain development and function.[1] The signs and symptoms of untreated or late-treated PKU can vary, depending on the clinical phenotype and include neurodevelopmental delay, mental retardation, impaired cognitive function, microcephaly, and neuromotor disorders.[1,4-7] Older children and adults with PKU can have behavioral problems, eczema, decreased measured intelligence quotients (IQ), and decreased exec-

From the Klinik für Kinder-und Jugendmedizin Reutlingen, Klinikum am Steinenberg, Reutlingen, Germany (F.T.); Division of Genetics, Children's Memorial Hospital, Chicago, IL (B.B.); Division of Medical Genetics, Department of Pediatrics, University of Utah, Salt Lake City, UT (N.L.); Hospital Ramón y Cajal, Madrid, Spain (M.C.); Emory University School of Medicine, Decatur, GA (D.G.); BioMarin Pharmaceutical Inc, Novato, CA (A.D., E.K.); UCLA Medical Center, Los Angeles, CA (E.C.); Washington University School of Medicine, St Louis, MO (D.G.); Children's Hospital & Research Center of Oakland, Oakland, CA (P.H.); The Permanente Medical Group, Sacramento, CA (M.L.); Instytut Matki i Dziecka, Warszawa, Poland (A.M.); Children's Hospital Los Angeles, Los Angeles, CA (L.R.); University of Pittsburgh School of Medicine, Pittsburgh, PA (J.V.); University of Minnesota Medical School, Minneapolis, MN (C.W.); University of Wisconsin Medical School, Madison, WI (J.W.); Statistics Collaborative Inc, Washington, DC (J.B.), and Charité University Medical Center, Berlin, Germany (J.H.).

*Additional members of the Sapropterin Study Group available at www.jpeds.com (Appendix).

This study has been registered on http://www.clinicaltrials.gov under the trial number NCT00272792.

Supported by BioMarin Pharmaceutical Inc, whose physician-scientists and staff had a significant role in study design, collection, analysis, and interpretation of data and the writing of the manuscript.

Submitted for publication Jan 13, 2008; last revision received Sep 15, 2008; accepted Nov 19, 2008.

Reprint requests: Prof Friedrich Trefz, Klinik für Kinder-und Jugendmedizin, Reutlingen Klinikum am Steinenberg, Steinenbergstrasse 31, Reutlingen D-72764, Germany. E-mail: ftrefz@ramedis.de

0022-3476/$ - see front matter

Copyright © 2009 Mosby Inc. All rights reserved.

10.1016/j.jpeds.2008.11.040

AE	Adverse event	Phe	Phenylalanine
ANOVA	Analysis of variance	PKU	Phenylketonuria
IQ	Intelligence quotient	SAE	Serious adverse event
PAH	Phenylalanine hydroxylase	SOC	System order class

700

utive function if Phe is uncontrolled later in life.[8-10] Based on these findings, a National Institutes of Health Consensus Panel has recommended maintaining control of blood Phe levels for life.[9]

Dietary restriction of Phe intake has been the treatment of choice to reduce Phe levels for more than 40 years and has led to the prevention of severe intellectual dysfunction in patients with PKU.[1,9] Even with this success, some patients have difficulty complying with the highly restricted medical diet that is required. The Phe-free protein formula included in the diet to provide daily protein requirements has an odd taste and odor, and many patients find it unpalatable.[11] As a result, adhering to the PKU diet is extremely challenging, resulting in a high rate of treatment noncompliance[12] that increases with age.[13,14]

Dietary Phe restriction has prevented severe mental deficiency, but many studies suggest that the intellectual outcomes of patients with PKU managed using a Phe-restricted diet are not optimal.[1,15] Well-controlled patients have IQs that are 5 to 7 points lower than their unaffected siblings, although generally within the normal range of 92 to 102.[16] These deficits are most likely caused by a combination of inconsistent compliance and nutritional deficiencies introduced with artificial diets.[1,15] In addition, when early-treated patients with PKU lessen dietary Phe control as teenagers or adults, they often suffer the consequences of neurological problems including deficits in executive functioning[17]; problems in school[18]; increased use of medications to treat attention-deficit hyperactivity disorder[19]; and problems with social integration.[20]

In view of the inconvenience and suboptimal outcomes of dietary management, there is a need for PKU treatments that can lower blood Phe concentrations and increase Phe tolerance. Tetrahydrobiopterin (BH4), a cofactor for PAH, has been shown to increase residual PAH activity and partially restore oxidative metabolism of Phe in a significant proportion of patients with PKU.[21-23] Several reports and case series have shown that BH4 can successfully increase Phe tolerance and decrease blood Phe concentrations in BH4-responsive patients.[22-28]

A new pharmaceutical formulation of tetrahydrobiopterin or 6R-BH4, (herein referred to as sapropterin) has been developed as a once-daily oral therapy for PKU. A recent Phase III study of sapropterin in 89 subjects with PKU 8 years old and above showed that oral administration of 10 mg/kg/d significantly reduced elevated blood Phe levels and showed safety comparable to placebo.[29] Here, we report results from a double-blind, randomized, placebo-controlled trial to evaluate the efficacy and safety of sapropterin at 20 mg/kg/d in increasing Phe tolerance while maintaining blood Phe control in 4- to 12-year-old subjects with PKU who were following a Phe-restricted diet.

METHODS

Trial Overview

This randomized, double-blind, placebo-controlled, Phase III clinical trial was conducted in 2 parts. In Part 1, subjects with PKU on dietary Phe restriction were screened for sapropterin responsiveness by open-label once-daily oral treatment with sapropterin, 20 mg/kg/d for 8 days. Subjects who met a defined response level to sapropterin continued into Part 2 after a washout period of at least 1 week. Responsive subjects were randomized into Part 2 and studied for the ability of sapropterin, 20 mg/kg/d, to increase Phe tolerance and reduce blood Phe concentrations and to assess the safety of sapropterin.

Subjects and Protocol

Subjects were eligible to participate in the study if they were 4 to 12 years of age, had a diagnosis of PKU with PAH deficiency, an estimated Phe tolerance ≤1000 mg/d, were under dietary control with a Phe-restricted diet, as evidenced by a mean blood Phe concentration ≤480 μmol/L over the 6 months before study enrollment, and had a blood Phe concentration of ≤480 μmol/L at screening. Subjects were excluded if they had a history of organ transplantation, use of any investigational agent within 30 days before screening, serum alanine aminotransferase levels of more than twice the upper limit of normal, concurrent disease that might interfere with participation (including untreated neuropsychiatric disorders), a requirement for treatment with any drug that inhibits folate synthesis, concurrent use of levodopa, or a diagnosis of primary BH4 deficiency.

Written informed consent was obtained for all subjects, either from a parent or guardian, and subjects gave written assent when appropriate. The study was approved by local Institutional Review Boards and Ethics Committees, and was conducted in accordance with the US Code of Federal Regulations for clinical research studies, the International Conference on Harmonization Guidelines for Good Clinical Practice and the Declaration of Helsinki. This study has been registered on http://www.clinicaltrials.gov under the trial number NCT00272792.

Study enrollment began in February 2006; the last assessment was performed in November 2006. Eligible subjects entered Part 1 and received an open-label, 8-day course of oral sapropterin, 20 mg/kg/d, once daily. Responders were arbitrarily defined as those who achieved a ≥30% reduction in blood Phe concentrations between day 1 (before sapropterin treatment) and day 8, had a blood Phe concentration of ≤300 μmol/L on day 8, and were eligible to enter Part 2. The ≤300 μmol/L criterion was included to ensure that subjects had a sufficiently low Phe level to allow for potential increases in Phe supplementation without exceeding the control guideline. Subjects who did not meet responder criteria were withdrawn from further participation and had a safety assessment performed 4 weeks after their last visit in Part 1.

After a washout period (no study drug) of ≥1 week, responders from Part 1 were randomized (3:1) to receive a 10-week course of sapropterin, 20 mg/kg/d, or placebo tablets containing only excipients, once daily. To ensure balance in the severity of PKU between the groups, randomization to treatment group was stratified by "high" or "low," using the average of the blood Phe concentration values available during the preceding 6 months (<300 or ≥300 μmol/L). Randomization was performed by a computer program and interactive voice-response system using block sizes of 4; the block sizes were not divulged to the study sponsor or investigators until the study was completed.

Subjects were instructed to maintain a stable, Phe-restricted diet throughout the study, monitored by diaries kept for 3 days of each week containing a record of weighed or measured amounts of all food and drinks ingested, including medical foods. Dietary records were reviewed by a qualified nutritionist at each site and analyzed by a central, independent, expert nutrition service (Nutrition and Diet Services; Portland, Oregon), both blinded to treatment assignment.

Beginning at the week 3 visit of Part 2, Phe supplements, in the form of nonfat dried milk powder (Carnation Non-fat Dry Milk with Vitamin A, 1.703 g Phe per 100 g of powder)[30] or dried egg white powder (Deb El Just Whites Egg Whites, 5.181 g Phe per 100 g of powder)[30] were added or removed at biweekly intervals based on the blood Phe concentrations from the previous week using a defined algorithm (Table I; available at www.jpeds.com). The maximum Phe supplement that could be prescribed during the study was 50 mg/kg/d, based on the rules for increases at each step (Table I). The Phe supplement amount was calculated as mg per kg of ideal body weight per day because it would have been difficult to use an absolute mg amount of Phe given the wide age and size range of the pediatric group of subjects included in this study. Subjects with a blood Phe concentration of ≥1200 μmol/L in 2 consecutive weekly blood samples were instructed to discontinue study drug treatment and receive dietary counseling. At the week 10 visit, sapropterin and Phe supplements were discontinued and a week 14 follow-up visit was scheduled.

Sapropterin was supplied as tablets containing 100 mg sapropterin dihydrochloride (77 mg of sapropterin) and excipient. Subjects received 20 mg/kg/d doses of sapropterin dihydrochloride. Doses were rounded (up or down) to the nearest 100 mg and administered once daily each morning, generally before breakfast. Tablets were dissolved in 120 to 240 mL of water or apple juice and the solution was administered within 30 minutes. Sapropterin and placebo tablets had similar taste and appearance.

Assessments

Blood samples were drawn 2.5 to 5 hours after a meal at screening, on days 1 (before treatment) and 8 of Part 1, and at weekly intervals from Part 2 week 0 (before treatment) to week 10. Blood (whole blood, plasma, or dry blood spots, depending on the laboratory) Phe concentrations were measured only in local laboratories that participated in a quality assurance program conducted by the metabolic laboratory at the Mayo Clinic, Rochester, Minnesota. The method used for each patient was consistent throughout the study.

Medical and dietary history was obtained at screening. Use of concomitant medications, vital signs, and weight were recorded at screening and at days 1 and 8 of Part 1, and weekly during Part 2. A physical examination and laboratory tests (chemistries, hematology, and urinalysis performed in a central laboratory) were performed at screening and at days 1 and 8 of Part 1, and at the visits in weeks 0, 2, 6, 10, and 14 of Part 2. Adverse events (AEs) were evaluated for severity, seriousness, and relationship to study drug.

The efficacy endpoint for Part 1 was the proportion of subjects who were classified as responders: subjects who on day 8 had a blood Phe concentration of ≤300 μmol/L and a reduction in blood Phe concentration of ≥30% as compared with day 1.

The primary efficacy endpoint for Part 2 was the daily Phe supplement tolerated by the sapropterin group at week 10 compared with week 0 (ie, 0 mg/kg/d). The Phe supplement tolerated was defined as the cumulative increase or decrease in Phe supplement prescribed in Part 2 at the last visit at which the subject had adequate blood Phe control, defined as a blood Phe concentration <360 μmol/L. The last visit at which the subject was under adequate blood Phe control may have occurred before week 10 if a later supplement increase led to a Phe level above 360 μmol/L. There are established guidelines for optimal ranges of blood Phe concentrations for patients with PKU, with acceptable upper and lower limits varying across different countries[1,9,31,32] and even among treatment centers within the United States.[31] The National Institutes of Health recommends maintaining blood Phe concentrations between 120 and 360 μmol/L.[9,33] Therefore, in this study, adequate blood Phe control was defined as a concentration of ≤360 μmol/L.

Secondary efficacy endpoints for Part 2 were the difference in blood Phe concentrations in the sapropterin group between week 0 (before dosing) and week 3 (before Phe supplementation) and the comparison of the sapropterin and placebo groups in the amount of Phe supplement tolerated at week 10.

The independent nutritionist used a proprietary program for diet analysis. Nutrient data were obtained from the US Department of Agriculture, Agricultural Research Service 2004 USDA National Nutrient Database for Standard Reference, Release 17,[30] and data supplied by manufacturers or available on food packages. For European products, data supplied by the subject, site dietician, or manufacturer's websites were used. When not provided, amino acid values were imputed as a percentage of protein. To maintain consistency and accuracy in data entry, one person entered diet data for a single subject over the span of the study and a different person reviewed the entry; both individuals remained blinded to study group assignment.

Statistical Analyses

Assuming a mean difference in Phe supplement tolerated of 17.5 mg/kg/d with the SD of 16.0 mg/kg/d (estimated on the basis of a literature review)[24,26] in the sapropterin group during Part 2, a sample size of 30 subjects receiving sapropterin would provide 99% power to detect a significant increase in Phe intake with a two-sided type I error rate = 0.05. Enrollment in Part 1 was continued until 50 sapropterin-responsive subjects were identified by responder screening.

For Part 1 (screening), all subjects who received at least 1 dose of study drug and had both day 1 and day 8 blood Phe concentrations measured were included in the efficacy analysis. Blood Phe concentrations for days 1 and 8 were compared for each subject. Those who were responders were eligible for Part 2.

For Part 2 (double-blind portion), all subjects who received at least 1 dose of study drug were included in the analyses of Phe supplement tolerated at week 10, regardless of treatment status at the week 10 visit. The total daily Phe supplement prescribed up until the last adjustment at which the subject had adequate blood Phe control (blood Phe concentration <360 μmol/L) was used. The safety analyses included all subjects who received at least one dose of study drug during either Part 1 or Part 2.

The primary efficacy endpoint for Part 2 was a comparison of the amount of Phe supplement tolerated at week 10 with the Phe supplement at baseline (0 mg/kg/d) for the sapropterin treatment group using a 1-sample t test. For a secondary endpoint, the sapropterin and placebo groups were compared with respect to the amount of Phe supplement tolerated at week 10 by a 2-way analysis of variance (ANOVA) model stratified by blood Phe concentration in the 6 months before Part 1. A second secondary endpoint was an analysis of the difference in blood Phe concentrations in the sapropterin group between the week 0 and the week 3 visits of Part 2 before Phe supplementation. This was assessed using a 1-sample t test with subjects acting as their own controls. A longitudinal model with weekly blood Phe measurements as the response variable and treatment group, visit, and baseline blood Phe concentration (average of measurements at screening, day 1 of Part 1 and week 0 of Part 2) as covariates was used to compare the treatment groups with respect to the supplementary analysis of mean change in weekly blood Phe concentration. Descriptive statistics were used for the supplementary analyses of mean change in weekly blood Phe concentrations and the daily Phe supplement prescribed, and for reporting AEs.

RESULTS

Screening and Subject Characteristics

In total, 117 subjects were screened in 15 centers across Europe and the United States, and 90 subjects (39 females, 51 males; mean [SD] age, 7.3 [2.5] years) were enrolled in Part 1 of the study and received at least 1 dose of sapropterin. Of these, 89 subjects also had blood Phe concentration recorded for day 8. Of the 50/89 (56%) who met responder criteria, 46 subjects were randomized in Part 2, and 45 subjects received at least 1 dose of either sapropterin (33 subjects) or placebo (12 subjects); 1 subject who was randomized to the sapropterin group did not return for the week 0 visit and therefore did not receive any study drug in Part 2 and was not included in the analyses. Four responders did not progress to Part 2 for various reasons unrelated to safety. The baseline demographic and physical characteristics were generally similar in the 2 groups (Table II).

Mean Phe levels (SD) in the 6 months before enrollment and the number of subjects in the stratum below 300 μmol/L were similar between the 2 groups (Table II). Dietary Phe intake (SD) at baseline week 0 was 16.8 (7.6) mg/kg/d for the sapropterin group or a mean of 511 mg/d and 16.3 (8.4) mg/kg/d or a mean of 450 mg/d for the placebo group. All subjects qualified as subjects with PKU (not mild HPA) based on the degree of dietary Phe restriction required to maintain Phe control.

The 50 responders in Part 1 experienced a decrease in mean (SD) blood Phe from 317.0 (173.2) μmol/L on day 1 to 108.1 (70.2) μmol/L on day 8. The mean (SD) reduction in blood Phe concentration from day 1 to day 8 was 209.0 (138.6) μmol/L and the mean (SD) percent change in blood Phe concentrations was 64.0% (17.5%). The mean (SD) blood Phe concentration of non-responders in Part 1 did not change: 234.3 (185.6) μmol/L on day 1 compared with 263.7 (171.1) μmol/L on day 8. Two subjects showed a reduction of ≥30% in blood Phe concentration during Part 1 but did not meet criteria for participation in Part 2 because they did not have blood Phe concentrations of ≤300 μmol/L on day 8.

Efficacy

During Part 2, subjects were randomized 3:1 to receive sapropterin at 20 mg/kg or placebo once per day, and all subjects were asked to maintain their PKU diet unchanged. The Phe supplement dose was adjusted every other week to determine the maximal tolerated Phe supplement achievable while maintaining good Phe control the week after each change. Over the 10-week period, subjects in the sapropterin

Table II. Demographics and physical characteristics of sapropterin-responsive subjects enrolled in Part 2 of the study

Characteristic	Sapropterin (n = 33)	Placebo (n = 12)
Age (y), mean (SD)	7.7 (2.8)	7.1 (2.0)
Sex, n (%) female	13 (39)	6 (50)
Weight (kg), mean (SD)	30.4 (9.8)	27.6 (8.0)
Body mass index (kg/m^2) mean (SD)	17.9 (2.3)	17.3 (2.2)
Blood Phe level (μmol/L) over prior 6 months, mean (SD)	314 (107)	303 (74)
Blood Phe level (μmol/L) over prior 6 months, range	112-474	176-447
Mean blood Phe <300 μmol/L over prior 6 months, n (%)	16 (48)	5 (42)
Baseline dietary Phe intake at week 0 (mg/kg/d), mean (SD)	16.3 (8.4)*	16.8 (7.6)†

*n = 30; †n = 9.

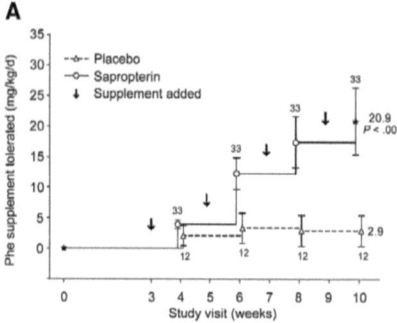

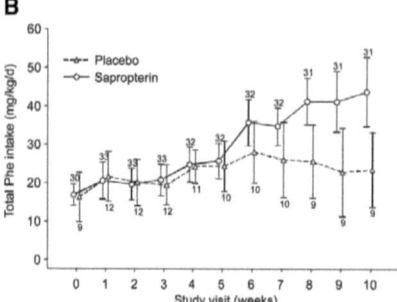

Figure. **A,** Total phenylalanine (Phe) supplement tolerated by subjects receiving sapropterin and placebo. Mean (95% CI) Phe total supplement tolerated (while the subject was under adequate blood Phe control, <360 μmol/L), by visit (last observation carried forward, where the daily Phe supplement tolerated at the last visit at which the subject was under adequate blood Phe control was used). The primary efficacy analysis compared the values before and after treatment in the sapropterin group, indicated by a star, using a 1-sample *t* test. Downward arrows indicate the weeks at which supplement could be increased for both groups, and the increase supplement was deemed tolerated by a Phe level assessed at the next week's visit. The numbers below the confidence limits are the numbers of subjects whose data is included in that assessment. **B,** Total mean Phe intake in subjects receiving sapropterin and placebo. Total Phe intake (95% CI) is shown as calculated by adding dietary Phe intake from diet histories to the Phe supplement taken for sapropterin and placebo. The total Phe taken at any week may include Phe taken but not tolerated based on the Phe level measured in subsequent weeks.

group (n = 33) tolerated a mean (SD) Phe supplement of 20.9 (15.4) mg/kg/d (95 % CI: 15.4 to 26.4) (*P* < .001 vs 0 mg/kg/d at week 0; Figure). Total Phe intake (dietary Phe intake plus total Phe supplement taken) at week 10 reached 43.8 (24.6) mg/kg/d in the sapropterin group (*P* < .0001 vs baseline), an approximate doubling in Phe taken (Figure). The sapropterin group had a mean (SD) Phe level of 340 (235) μmol/L at week 10.

The placebo group had an increase of 2.9 mg/kg/d in tolerated Phe supplement during the 10-week period (Figure), and a modest increase in total Phe intake from 16.3 (8.4) mg/kg/d to 23.5 (12.6) mg/kg/d at week 10 that was not statistically significant (Figure). The placebo group had an elevated mean (SD) Phe level of 461 (235) μmol/L at week 10.

To compare the Phe supplement tolerated by the sapropterin group with that tolerated by the placebo group, an ANOVA model was used. As estimated by the ANOVA model, the mean ± SE of Phe supplement tolerated by subjects receiving sapropterin (21.0 ± 2.3 mg/kg/d) was significantly greater than the amount tolerated by those receiving placebo (3.3 ± 3.9 mg/kg/d). The adjusted mean ± SE of the treatment group difference was 17.7 ± 4.5 mg/kg/d, corresponding to a 95% CI of 9 to 27 (*P* < .001).

When evaluating the outcomes of individual subjects, there was a range of Phe supplement tolerance achieved within the sapropterin group. Over the 10-week period, 12 of 33 subjects (36%) in the sapropterin group tolerated an increase of 10 mg/kg/d or less of Phe supplement, 10 subjects (30%) tolerated an increase of 11 to 30 mg/kg/d, and 11 subjects (33%) tolerated an increase of 31 to 50 mg/kg/d. In contrast, no subject in the placebo group (n = 12) tolerated an increase of more than 10 mg/kg/d of Phe supplement during the 10 weeks, and 7 of 12 subjects (58%) could not tolerate any Phe supplement, compared with 5 subjects (15%) in the sapropterin group.

In the first 3 weeks of Part 2, before receiving Phe supplementation, mean blood Phe concentrations decreased significantly between weeks 0 and 3 in the sapropterin group. The mean (SD) blood Phe concentration in the sapropterin group decreased from 275.7 (135.2) μmol/L at week 0 before treatment to 111.5 (75.7) μmol/L at week 1 after initiation of sapropterin treatment and 2 weeks before Phe supplementation, and remained reduced at weeks 2 (115.9 [96.8] μmol/L; n = 32) and 3 (127.2 [89.6] μmol/L; n = 33) before Phe supplementation. The sapropterin group had a mean (SD) decrease of -148.5 (134.2) μmol/L (95% CI: [-196 to -101]) in Phe blood concentrations between weeks 0 and 3 before Phe supplementation (data not shown), which differed significantly from 0 μmol/L (1-sample *t* test: *P* < .001).

In the placebo group, the mean (SD) change in blood Phe level (-96.6 [243.6] μmol/L) was not significantly different from 0 μmol/L (95% CI: -251 to 58; *P* = .20) due to a large degree of variability. The longitudinal model showed an estimated mean (±SE) difference in blood Phe concentrations between the sapropterin and placebo groups at week 3 of -135.2 (±26.9) μmol/L (*P* < .001). Given that the blood Phe levels were required to be low at screening, the change represents a decrease that is incremental to ongoing dietary restriction.

Safety

In Part 1, 52 AEs were reported for 28 of 90 subjects (31%). Abdominal pain was the only AE reported by more than 5% (5/90, 6%) of subjects; headache was reported by 4

Table III. Adverse events with highest incidence (>5% subjects in the sapropterin group) during Part 2 of the study

Adverse event	Sapropterin, n (%) (n = 33)	Placebo, n (%) (n = 12)
Rhinorrhea	7 (21)	0 (0)
Headache	7 (21)	1 (8)
Cough	5 (15)	0 (0)
Pharyngolaryngeal pain	4 (12)	1 (8)
Diarrhea	4 (12)	0 (0)
Vomiting	4 (12)	0 (0)
Abdominal pain	3 (9)	1 (8)
Contusion	3 (9)	1 (8)
Nasal congestion	3 (9)	0 (0)
Pyrexia	3 (9)	2 (17)
Decreased appetite	2 (6)	0 (0)
Erythema	2 (6)	0 (0)
Excoriation	2 (6)	0 (0)
Lymphadenopathy	2 (6)	0 (0)
Streptococcal infection	2 (6)	2 (17)
Toothache	2 (6)	0 (0)
Upper respiratory tract infection	2 (6)	1 (8)

subjects (4%), and all other AEs were reported only infrequently. The investigators considered 23 of the 52 AEs (44%) reported by 15 subjects (17%) to be possibly or probably related to sapropterin, with gastrointestinal disorders (eg, abdominal pain, nausea, and diarrhea) having the highest incidence of possibly or probably related AEs of any system organ class (SOC). No serious AE (SAE) was reported during Part 1.

In Part 2, a total of 128 AEs were reported for 34 (76%) of the 45 subjects, regardless of relatedness to treatment. AEs reported most frequently (>5% of subjects receiving sapropterin) are shown in Table III. Headaches appeared to be more common in the treated group.

AEs considered by the investigator to be possibly related to study treatment were reported by similar proportions of subjects in the sapropterin and placebo groups (27% and 25%, respectively). SAEs were reported for 2 subjects (1 report of appendicitis in the placebo group and 1 report of streptococcal infection in the sapropterin group), but neither was considered possibly or probably related to the study drug.

During both parts of the study, there were no severe AEs or AEs that led to withdrawal of study drug or study participation. Analyses of clinical laboratory variables, vital signs measurements, and physical examinations did not reveal clinically significant abnormalities. Mild to moderate neutropenia (absolute neutrophil count <1500 cells per μL) was noted in 7 of 33 (21%) subjects in the sapropterin group and 2 of 12 (17%) subjects in the placebo group. No discernible pattern of decrease in neutrophil count was noted, and no subjects had a level less than 500 cells per μL. Neutropenic events tended to occur in subjects with lower white blood counts at baseline. No events were recorded as related to treatment. None of the neutropenic events were serious or associated with increased risk of infection.

Low Phe levels occurred more often in the treated group, as might be expected, due to the effect of the drug on lowering Phe and the requirement of controlled Phe levels at baseline. Among the 45 subjects included in the Part 2 safety analysis, 13 in the sapropterin group (22 occurrences) and only 1 in the placebo group (1 occurrence at week 4 of Part 2) had a blood Phe concentration below 26 μmol/L (lower limit of age-related normal range at the Mayo Clinic Laboratory). In the sapropterin group, 6 subjects had low blood Phe concentrations (<26 μmol/L) before the addition of the protocol-defined Phe supplement at week 3, 3 had low blood Phe concentrations at week 4, and 1 had low blood Phe concentrations at weeks 6 and 7. All low blood Phe levels were transient, no subject had low blood Phe concentrations during the last 3 weeks of the study, no subject in the sapropterin group finished the study with a low blood Phe concentration, and no adverse symptoms of low blood Phe concentrations were noted in any subject.

DISCUSSION

This international, multicenter, randomized, placebo-controlled trial demonstrated that daily dosing with sapropterin led to significant increases in Phe tolerance, while maintaining blood Phe control. Subjects with PKU who are responsive to sapropterin have a reduction in blood Phe levels and improved Phe tolerance, and could increase their dietary Phe intake and maintain equal or better Phe control. Sapropterin treatment increased Phe tolerance significantly, representing an approximate doubling for the mean Phe taken and for 30% of the subjects, the increase reached 30 to 50 mg/kg/d. An analysis of diet prescriptions would suggest that size of mean increase in Phe tolerance could allow an average responsive subject to maintain control while eating regular versions of PKU-restricted foods, reducing the required Phe-free formula intake by two-thirds. For the most responsive subjects achieving 30 to 50 mg/kg/d of supplement tolerated, the total of about 40 to 70 mg/kg/d would allow a more normal diet. The introduction of natural protein sources into the diet could also provide better nutritional balance, including more normal levels of micronutrients, which are essential for satisfactory growth and development in children.[28]

Our results are consistent with several studies that have reported improved Phe tolerance in patients with PKU with treatment using other formulations of BH4.[22,24-28] In a study extending up to 18 months, 7 children with mild PKU who received sapropterin at least doubled their protein intake, and some were able to discontinue the Phe-free protein supplement entirely.[27] In another report, Phe tolerance improved sufficiently in 11 of 14 children with mild/moderate PKU to allow gradual reduction and, in some cases, discontinuation of Phe-free protein supplement over 1 year of treatment with BH4.[28] In a small open-label study of 5 children with mild PKU who were treated for approximately 30 weeks with 7.1 to 10.7 mg/kg daily of sapropterin, mean total daily

Phe tolerance increased significantly from 19 mg/kg/d to 61 mg/kg/d.[22] Finally, 5 infants with severe classic PKU had a sustained response for up to 2 years of treatment with BH4, 20 mg/kg/d, allowing substantial easing of dietary restrictions; total daily Phe intake increased from 18 to 19 mg/kg/d, to 30 to 80 mg/kg/d over the treatment period.[26]

In the present study, sapropterin treatment significantly reduced blood Phe concentrations in subjects following a Phe-restricted diet and whose blood Phe concentration was considered to be under control at the time of enrollment. For some subjects, the blood Phe concentration fell below 26 μmol/L before supplementation. These low Phe blood concentrations were transient and responded to increases in Phe supplement according to the study protocol. However, it is important to monitor blood Phe concentrations closely in subjects with PKU treated with sapropterin, and the dietary Phe intake may need to be adjusted on the basis of blood Phe concentrations to ensure that periods of low Phe levels are not prolonged.[34]

The conclusions of the current study are limited to children with PKU, responsive to sapropterin, with blood Phe concentrations controlled on a Phe-restricted diet. At baseline, patients in the sapropterin and placebo groups tolerated Phe at a level of 16.8 and 16.3 mg/kg/d, respectively. Such a low Phe tolerance has previously been observed in 5-year old patients with classical PKU.[35] However, this study was not designed to evaluate whether BH4 treatment was more effective in patients with milder PKU than in patients with classic PKU, which may be the case. Existing data from other studies indicate that sapropterin can lead to clinically significant reductions in blood Phe concentrations in individuals with PKU not adequately controlled on diet therapy.[25-28]

This study indicates that sapropterin has an acceptable safety profile in subjects with PKU as young as 4 years old, and in doses up to 20 mg/kg/d. There was a moderate increase in the number of AEs in the gastrointestinal disorders SOC among those receiving sapropterin compared with placebo. As an acidic product, it could be hypothesized that sapropterin might cause irritation of the gastrointestinal tract if not taken with food.

One other difference between the treatment groups in the nervous system disorders SOC was an apparently higher incidence of headache in the sapropterin group, a difference that would disappear if the placebo group had reported one more headache. It is important to recognize that with a 3:1 ratio for randomization, the placebo group is relatively small, making it difficult to draw firm conclusions on causality in this study. A larger double-blind, placebo-controlled study of sapropterin in subjects 8 years and above also found a safety profile similar to placebo and no increased incidence of headaches.[29] As for all new therapeutic agents, continued long-term monitoring of AEs will further define the safety profile of sapropterin in the treatment of BH4-responsive patients with PKU.

In conclusion, treatment with sapropterin (20 mg/kg/d as sapropterin dihydrochloride) in BH4-responsive children with PKU who are controlled on a Phe-restricted diet reduces blood Phe concentrations and increases Phe tolerance. These results suggest that sapropterin treatment may allow a subset of subjects with PKU to increase intake of dietary protein and reduce the need for Phe-free protein supplements and still achieve prescribed blood Phe control goals of therapy.

The authors would like to thank Stuart Swiedler MD, PhD (former Senior Vice President of Clinical Affairs for BioMarin Pharmaceutical, Inc.), and Harvey Levy, MD (member of the National PKU Advisory Board and consultant for BioMarin Pharmaceutical, Inc.), for their assistance in the design and execution of the study. The authors also thank Dr Phillippa Curran (supported by BioMarin Pharmaceutical Inc. and Merck Serono S.A.-Geneva) for her assistance in the preparation of this manuscript.

REFERENCES

1. Scriver CR, Kaufman S. Hyperphenylalaninemia: phenylalanine hydroxylase deficiency. In: Scriver CR, Beaudet AL, Sly WS, Valle D, editors. Metabolic and Molecular Bases of Inherited Disease. New York: McGraw-Hill; 2001. p. 1667-724.
2. Phenylalanine Hydroxylase Locus Knowledgebase. http://www.PAHdb.mcgill.ca. 2007.
3. Loeber JG. Neonatal screening in Europe; the situation in 2004. J Inherit Metab Dis 2007;30:430-8.
4. Antshel KM, Waisbren SE. Timing is everything: executive functions in children exposed to elevated levels of phenylalanine. Neuropsychology 2003;17:458-68.
5. Diamond A, Prevor MB, Callender G, Druin DP. Prefrontal cortex cognitive deficits in children treated early and continuously for PKU. Monogr Soc Res Child Dev 1997;62:i-v, 1-208.
6. Krause W, Epstein C, Averbook A, Dembure P, Elsas L. Phenylalanine alters the mean power frequency of electroencephalograms and plasma L-dopa in treated patients with phenylketonuria. Pediatr Res 1986;20:1112-6.
7. Moyle JJ, Fox AM, Arthur M, Bynevelt M, Burnett JR. Meta-analysis of neuropsychological symptoms of adolescents and adults with PKU. Neuropsychol Rev 2007;17:91-101.
8. Brumm VL, Azen C, Moats RA, Stern AM, Broomand C, Nelson MD, et al. Neuropsychological outcome of subjects participating in the PKU adult collaborative study: a preliminary review. J Inherit Metab Dis 2004;27:549-66.
9. National Institutes of Health Consensus Development Panel. National Institutes of Health Consensus Development Conference statement: Phenylketonuria: screening and management, October 16-18, 2000. Pediatrics 2001;108:972-82.
10. Paine RS. Variability in manifestations of untreated patients with phenylketonuria. Pediatrics 1957;20:290-302.
11. Rohr FJ, Munier AW, Levy HL. Acceptability of a new modular protein substitute for the dietary treatment of phenylketonuria. J Inherit Metab Dis 2001;24:623-30.
12. Rylance G. Outcome of early detected and early treated phenylketonuria patients. Postgrad Med J 1989;65(Suppl 2):S7-9.
13. Fisch RO. Comments on diet and compliance in phenylketonuria. Eur J Pediatr 2000;159(Suppl 2):S142-4.
14. Walter JH, White FJ, MacDonald A, Rylance G, Boneh A, Francis DE, et al. How practical are recommendations for dietary control in phenylketonuria? Lancet 2002;360:55-7.
15. Smith I, Beasley MG, Ades AE. Intelligence and quality of dietary treatment in phenylketonuria. Arch Dis Child 1990;65:472-8.
16. Azen C, Koch R, Friedman E, Wenz E, Fishler K. Summary of findings from the United States Collaborative Study of children treated for phenylketonuria. Eur J Pediatr 1996;155(Suppl 1):S29-32.
17. White DA, Nortz MJ, Mandernach T, Huntington K, Steiner RD. Deficits in memory strategy use related to prefrontal dysfunction during early development: evidence from children with phenylketonuria. Neuropsychology 2001;15:221-9.
18. Gassio R, Fuste E, Lopez-Sala A, Artuch R, Vilaseca MA, Campistol J. School performance in early and continuously treated phenylketonuria. Pediatr Neurol 2005;33:267-71.
19. Arnold GL, Vladutiu CJ, Orlowski CC, Blakely EM, DeLuca J. Prevalence of stimulant use for attentional dysfunction in children with phenylketonuria. J Inherit Metab Dis 2004;27:137-43.
20. Bhat M, Haase C, Lee PJ. Social outcome in treated individuals with inherited metabolic disorders: UK study. J Inherit Metab Dis 2005;28:825-30.
21. Kure S, Hou D, Ohura T, Iwamoto H, Suzuki S, Sugiyama N, et al. Tetrahydrobiopterin-responsive phenylalanine hydroxylase deficiency. J Pediatr 1999;135:375-8.
22. Muntau AC, Röschinger W, Habich M, Demmelmair H, Hoffmann B, Sommerhoff CP, et al. Tetrahydrobiopterin as an alternative treatment for mild phenylketonuria. N Engl J Med 2002;347:2122-32.

23. Zurflüh MR, Zschocke J, Lindner M, Feillet F, Chery C, Burlina A, et al. Molecular genetics of tetrahydrobiopterin-responsive phenylalanine hydroxylase deficiency. Hum Mutat 2008;29:167-75.
24. Trefz FK, Scheible D, Frauendienst-Egger G, Korall H, Blau N. Long-term treatment of patients with mild and classical phenylketonuria by tetrahydrobiopterin. Mol Genet Metab 2005;86(Suppl 1):S75-80.
25. Shintaku H, Kure S, Ohura T, Okano Y, Ohwada M, Sugiyama N, et al. Long-term treatment and diagnosis of tetrahydrobiopterin-responsive hyperphenylalaninemia with a mutant phenylalanine hydroxylase gene. Pediatr Res 2004;55:425-30.
26. Hennermann JB, Buhrer C, Blau N, Vetter B, Monch E. Long-term treatment with tetrahydrobiopterin increases phenylalanine tolerance in children with severe phenotype of phenylketonuria. Mol Genet Metab 2005;86(Suppl 1):S86-90.
27. Belanger-Quintana A, Garcia MJ, Castro M, Desviat LR, Perez B, Mejia B, et al. Spanish BH4-responsive phenylalanine hydroxylase-deficient patients: evolution of seven patients on long-term treatment with tetrahydrobiopterin. Mol Genet Metab 2005;86(Suppl 1):S61-6.
28. Lambruschini N, Perez-Duenas B, Vilaseca MA, Mas A, Artuch R, Gassio R, et al. Clinical and nutritional evaluation of phenylketonuric patients on tetrahydrobiopterin monotherapy. Mol Genet Metab 2005;86(Suppl 1):S54-60.
29. Levy HL, Milanowski A, Chakrapani A, Cleary M, Lee P, Trefz FK, et al; Sapropterin Research Group. Efficacy of sapropterin dihydrochloride (tetrahydrobiopterin, 6R-BH4) for reduction of phenylalanine concentration in patients with phenylketonuria: a phase III randomised placebo-controlled study. Lancet 2007; 370:504-510.
30. US Department of Agriculture ARS. USDA National Nutrient Database for Standard Reference, Release 17. Nutrient Data Laboratory Home Page, http://www.nal.usda.gov/fnic/foodcomp. 2004.
31. Wappner R, Cho S, Kronmal RA, Schuett V, Seashore MR. Management of phenylketonuria for optimal outcome: a review of guidelines for phenylketonuria management and a report of surveys of parents, patients, and clinic directors. Pediatrics 1999;104:e68.
32. Burgard P, Bremer HJ, Buhrdel P, Clemens PC, Monch E, Przyrembel H, et al. Rationale for the German recommendations for phenylalanine level control in phenylketonuria 1997. Eur J Pediatr 1999;158:46-54.
33. Phenylketonuria (PKU): screening and management. NIH Consensus Statement 2000;17:1-33.
34. Levy H, Burton B, Cederbaum S, Scriver C. Recommendations for evaluation of responsiveness to tetrahydrobiopterin (BH[4]) in phenylketonuria and its use in treatment. Mol Genet Metab 2007;92:287-91.
35. Güttler F. Hyperphenylalaninemia: diagnosis and classification of the various types of phenylalanine hydroxylase deficiency in childhood. Acta Paediatr Scand Suppl 1980;280:1-80.

50 Years Ago in The Journal of Pediatrics

TONSILLECTOMY DURING THE POLIOVIRUS SEASON

Greenberg M. J Pediatr 1959;54:722-4

In this editorial, Greenberg reviewed the response of the World Health Organization (WHO) as well as US opinion leaders in 1957 to the question: "Should there be relaxation of the prohibition of elective tonsillectomy and adenoidectomy (T&A) during the polio season (summer months in the US)?" Before the advent of the poliovirus vaccine, there was ample and distressing evidence indicating that performing T&A during the early stages of poliovirus infection increased the risk of bulbar disease. Enteroviruses, including polioviruses, colonize the pharynx as well as the lower gastrointestinal tract. Bulbar encephalitis occurring after T&A was thought to result from direct inoculation and extension of the virus from pharyngeal nerves. The Salk inactivated vaccine already had prevented thousands of cases of paralytic poliomyelitis and reduced epidemic disease by 1959, but several caveats regarding the vaccine's effect were relevant to the WHO's deliberation. First, it was well known that intestinal excretion and pharyngeal excretion occurred despite complete immunization. Second, early Salk vaccine was not uniformly potent. In 1958, 322 cases of paralytic poliomyelitis and 20 deaths occurred in individuals who had received 3 doses of Salk vaccine. Not surprisingly, the WHO upheld the recommendation to "prohibit" T&A during poliovirus season.

In reviewing this issue, Greenberg also called the reader's attention to a recent article by Bakwin[1] that not only raised considerable doubt regarding any advantages from the T&A operation, but also reported that between 1950 and 1955, 220 to 346 persons died each year as a direct effect of the operation in the United States.

Poliovirus aside, it would take another 20 years to reverse the tide of "routine" T&A. Now, after another 10 to 20 years of restraint, we are inching back toward ever-increasing indications and popularity for the procedure. This writer's experience with cases of bacterial meningitis and enteroviral bulbar encephalitis directly associated with T&A reminds us all that even though the poliomyelitis question is off the table in the United States (thanks to the eradication of endemic disease), T&A is not risk-free.

Sarah S. Long, MD
Section of Infectious Diseases
St Christopher's Hospital for Children
Philadelphia, Pennsylvania
10.1016/j.jpeds.2008.11.026

REFERENCES

1. Bakwin H. The tonsil-adenoidectomy enigma. J Pediatr 1958;52:339-61.

Table I. Phenylalanine (Phe) supplementation algorithm

Range of the week 2 blood Phe concentration (μmol/L)		Action
Low	High	
0	300	Increase Phe supplement by 5 mg/kg/d
301	480	No change in Phe supplement intake
481	Infinity	No change in Phe supplement intake and monitor blood Phe level at the next visit

Range of the blood Phe concentration at weeks 4, 6, and 8 (μmol/L)		Action at the next visit	
Low	High		
0	180	Increase Phe supplement by 15 mg/kg/d	
181	240	Increase Phe supplement by 10 mg/kg/d	
241	300	Increase Phe supplement by 5 mg/kg/d	
301	359	No change in Phe supplement intake	
360	Infinity	Did the subject have one or more previous Phe supplement increase(s)?	
		Yes ↓	No ↓
		Remove Phe supplement in the order that it was previously increased, beginning with the amount of the last increase	No change in Phe supplement intake
481	1199	1. If first occasion at this level, monitor blood Phe concentration at the next visit 2. If second occasion at this level, provide dietary counseling	
1200	Infinity	1. If first occasion at this level, provide dietary counseling and monitor blood Phe concentration at the next visit 2. If second occasion at this level, provide dietary counseling and terminate from study drug	

APPENDIX
SAPROPTERIN STUDY GROUP MEMBERS:

Barbara K Burton MD, Children's Memorial Hospital, Chicago, IL, USA; Eric A Crombez MD, UCLA Medical Center, Los Angeles, CA, USA; Dorothy K Grange MD, Washington School of Medicine, St Louis, MO, USA; Daniel J Gruskin MD, Emory University School of Medicine, Decatur, GA, USA; Paul Harmatz MD, Children's Hospital and Research Center of Oakland, Oakland, CA, USA; Julia B Hennermann MD, Charité University Medical Center, Berlin, Germany; Harvey L Levy, Children's Hospital of Boston, Boston, MA, USA; Mark H Lipson MD, The Permanente Medical Group, Sacramento, CA, USA; Nicola Longo MD, PhD, University of Utah, Salt Lake City, UT, USA; Mercedes Martinez-Pardo Casanova MD, Hospital Ramón y Cajal, Madrid, Spain; Andrzej Milanowski MD, PhD, Instytut Matki i Dziecka, Warszawa, Poland; Linda M Randolph MD, Children's Hospital Los Angeles, Los Angeles, CA, USA; Friedrich Trefz, Klinik für Kinder-und Jugendmedizin Reutlingen, Reutlingen, Germany; Jerry Vockley MD, PhD, University of Pittsburgh School of Medicine, Pittsburgh, PA, USA; Chester B Whitley PhD, MD, University of Minnesota Medical Center, Minneapolis, MN, USA; Jon A Wolff MD, University of Wisconsin Medical School, Madison, WI, USA.

2.5. PUBLIKATION 5: Burton BK, Nowacka M, **Hennermann JB**, Lipson M, Grange DK, Chakrapani A, Trefz F, Dorenbaum A, Imperiale M, Kim SS, Fernhoff PM. Safety of Extended Treatment with Sapropterin Dihydrochloride in Patients with Phenylketonuria: Results of a Phase 3b Study. 2011. Mol Genet Metab 103:315-322. DOI 10.1016/j.ymgme.2011.03.020

Reprinted from: Molecular Genetics and Metabolism 2011, Volume 103 (4), page 315-22, with permission from Elsevier Inc., 2011, provided by Copyright Clearance Center

Ziel dieser Studie war die Untersuchung der Sicherheit der Langzeittherapie mit Sapropterin bei BH4-responsiven Patienten mit PKU. Die Studie war eine multizentrische, multinationale Phase 3b-Open-Label-Anschlussstudie. Alle 111 Studienteilnehmer im Alter von 16,4 ± 10,2 Jahren (Spanne: 4-50 Jahre) hatten zuvor an einer Phase 3-Sapropterin-Studie teilgenommen. Die durchschnittliche Studienteilnahme betrug 659 ± 221 Tage, die gesamte Dauer der Sapropterin-Exposition bei allen Patienten 799 ± 238 Tage. Die durchschnittliche Sapropterin Dosis lag bei 16,2 ± 4,7 mg/kg/Tag.

Die meisten der unter Sapropterin beobachteten unerwünschten Ereignisse wurden als leicht oder mittelschwer und als nicht medikamentenassoziiert eingestuft. Zu den häufigsten möglicherweise medikamentenassoziierten unerwünschten Ereignissen zählten virale Gastroenteritiden, Erbrechen und Kopfschmerzen (jeweils 4,5%). Bei 7 Patienten traten schwerwiegende unerwünschte Ereignisse auf, von denen nur eines, ein gastroösophagealer Reflux, als möglicherweise medikamentenassoziiert klassifiziert wurde. 3 Patienten beendeten die Behandlung wegen möglicherweise medikamentenassoziierter unerwünschter Ereignisse. Diese waren Konzentrationsschwierigkeiten und Stimmungsschwankungen, Thrombozytopenie sowie intermittierende Diarrhoe. Bei 2 Patienten zeigte sich eine intermittierende Transaminasenerhöhung, bei 24 Patienten eine transiente nicht-behandlungsbedürftige Neutropenie (neutrophile Granulozyten <1.5×10^9/L) und bei 13 Patienten eine Thrombozytopenie, bei lediglich 4 davon mit Thrombozytenzahlen <100×10^9/L. Weitere Laborveränderungen ergaben sich bei den Studienteilnehmern nicht. Die Phe-Blutwerte blieben bei der Mehrzahl der Patienten unter Sapropterin-Therapie innerhalb des Zielbereiches.

Anhand dieser Studie konnte gezeigt werden, dass die Langzeittherapie mit Sapropterin in einer Dosierung von 5-20 mg/kg KG/Tag ein gutes Sicherheitsprofil aufweist und von den Patienten gut toleriert wird.

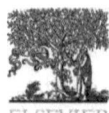 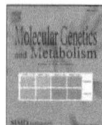

Molecular Genetics and Metabolism

journal homepage: www.elsevier.com/locate/ymgme

Safety of extended treatment with sapropterin dihydrochloride in patients with phenylketonuria: Results of a phase 3b study

Barbara K. Burton [a],*, Maria Nowacka [b], Julia B. Hennermann [c], Mark Lipson [d], Dorothy K. Grange [e], Anupam Chakrapani [f], Friedrich Trefz [g], Alex Dorenbaum [h], Michael Imperiale [i], Sun Sook Kim [i], Paul M. Fernhoff [j],1

[a] Children's Memorial Hospital, Chicago, IL, USA
[b] Instytut Matki I Dziecka, Warszawa, Poland
[c] Charité University Medical Center, Berlin, Germany
[d] Kaiser Permanente Medical Center, Sacramento, CA, USA
[e] Washington University School of Medicine, St. Louis, MO, USA
[f] Birmingham Children's Hospital, Birmingham, UK
[g] Klinik für Kinder-und Jugendmedizin Reutlingen, Reutlingen, Germany
[h] Previously BioMarin Pharmaceutical, Inc., Novato, CA, USA; Now Genentech, Inc., South San Francisco, CA, USA
[i] BioMarin Pharmaceutical, Inc., Novato, CA, USA
[j] Emory University School of Medicine, Decatur, GA, USA

ARTICLE INFO

Article history:
Received 2 February 2011
Received in revised form 24 March 2011
Accepted 24 March 2011
Available online 31 March 2011

Keywords:
6R-BH$_4$
Clinical trial
Phenylalanine
Phenylketonuria
Sapropterin
Tetrahydrobiopterin

ABSTRACT

Background: Phenylketonuria (PKU) results from impaired breakdown of phenylalanine (Phe) due to deficient phenylalanine hydroxylase (PAH) activity. Sapropterin dihydrochloride (sapropterin, Kuvan®) is the only US- and EU-approved pharmaceutical version of naturally occurring 6R-BH$_4$, the cofactor required for PAH activity. Sapropterin enhances residual PAH activity in sapropterin-responsive PKU patients and, in conjunction with dietary management, helps reduce blood Phe concentrations for optimal control. Approval was based on the positive safety and efficacy results of four international clinical studies, the longest of which was 22 weeks in duration.
Objective: To evaluate the safety of long-term treatment with sapropterin in PKU subjects who participated in previous Phase 3 sapropterin trials.
Methods: PKU-008 was designed as a Phase 3b, multicenter, multinational, open-label, 3-year extension trial to evaluate the long-term safety of sapropterin in patients with PKU who were classified as sapropterin responders and participated in prior Phase 3 sapropterin studies: 111 subjects aged 4–50 years completed prior studies and were subsequently enrolled in study PKU-008. Routine safety monitoring was performed at 3-month intervals and included adverse event reporting, blood Phe monitoring, clinical laboratory evaluations, physical examinations and vital sign measurements.
Results: Average exposure during PKU-008 was 658.7 ± 221.3 days (range, 56–953; median, 595). The average total duration of participation in multiple studies (PKU-001, PKU-003, PKU-004, and PKU-008; or PKU-006 and PKU-008) was 799.0 ± 237.5 days (range, 135-1151). The mean sapropterin dose was 16.2 ± 4.7 mg/kg/day. Most adverse events were considered unrelated to treatment, were mild or moderate in severity, and were consistent with prior studies of sapropterin. No age-specific differences were observed in adverse event reporting. Three subjects discontinued treatment due to adverse events that were considered possibly or probably related to study treatment (one each of difficulty concentrating, decreased platelet count, and intermittent diarrhea). No deaths were reported. Of seven reported serious adverse events, one was considered possibly related to study treatment (gastroesophageal reflux). There were no laboratory or physical examination abnormalities requiring medical interventions. For most subjects, blood Phe concentrations were consistently within target range, confirming the durability of response in subjects undergoing extended treatment with sapropterin.
Conclusion: Sapropterin treatment was found to be safe and well tolerated at doses of 5 to 20 mg/kg/day for an average exposure of 659 days. This study supports the safety and tolerability of sapropterin as long-term treatment for patients with PKU.

© 2011 Elsevier Inc. All rights reserved.

Abbreviations: 6R-BH$_4$, 6R-tetrahydrobiopterin; AE, adverse event; PKU, phenylketonuria; PAH, phenylalanine hydroxylase; Phe, phenylalanine; SAE, serious adverse event; ULN, upper limit of normal.
* Corresponding author at: Division of Genetics, Birth Defects, and Metabolism, Children's Memorial Hospital, 2300 North Childrens Plaza, Chicago, IL 60614, USA. Fax: +1 773 929 9565.
 E-mail address: bburton@childrensmemorial.org (B.K. Burton).
[1] For the Sapropterin Research Group.

1096-7192/$ – see front matter © 2011 Elsevier Inc. All rights reserved.
doi:10.1016/j.ymgme.2011.03.020

1. Introduction

Phenylketonuria (PKU) is a rare, autosomal recessive, metabolic disorder caused by mutations in the gene encoding phenylalanine hydroxylase (PAH) [1]. Impaired hydroxylation of phenylalanine (Phe), an essential amino acid solely obtainable through dietary sources, results in the toxic accumulation of Phe [1]; elevated blood Phe is the biochemical hallmark of PKU. Left untreated, PKU manifests in severe neurocognitive, neuropsychiatric, and neuromotor impairment [1,2]. Prior to publication of the 2000 NIH guidelines, PKU management strategies focused on strict control of blood Phe concentrations mainly during childhood [3]. Evidence-based review of the literature regarding suboptimal outcomes and relationship to elevated blood Phe concentrations for PKU patients in all age groups caused consensus groups to recommend that patients with PKU should maintain adequate control of blood Phe concentrations throughout their lives [3].

For the first approximately 40 years after initiation of routine screening of newborns for PKU, the only widespread treatment option available to control toxic Phe concentrations and prevent severe intellectual dysfunction in these patients was strict dietary restriction of Phe intake. Unfortunately, adherence with a Phe-restricted diet has historically been suboptimal [reviewed by Ref. 4]. In 1999, Kure et al. [5] demonstrated that orally administered 6R-tetrahydrobiopterin (6R-BH_4), an endogenous enzyme cofactor that is essential for PAH enzyme activity, effectively lowers blood Phe concentrations in a subset of PKU patients (further supported by subsequent studies [5–11]). In 2007 and 2008, respectively, the US and EU approved sapropterin dihydrochloride (sapropterin, Kuvan®), a pharmaceutical version of naturally occurring 6R-BH_4, as a new treatment option for reducing blood Phe concentrations in sapropterin-responsive PKU patients (≥4 years old in EU). Sapropterin, which can be used as a once-daily oral therapy in conjunction with dietary management, is the only drug that is approved for the treatment of PKU. Approval was based on positive safety and efficacy results of four international clinical studies [12–15]. The first three studies (PKU-001, PKU-003, and PKU-004) were conducted sequentially with the study population of the next being selected from the previous. Subjects in these studies were PKU patients ≥8 years old with poorly controlled hyperphenylalaninemia. PKU-001 was an open-label Phase 2 screening study that classified 96 of 485 patients as responders to sapropterin therapy (10 mg/kg/day), defined as a ≥30% reduction from baseline in blood Phe concentrations at the end of the 8-day study [12]. PKU-003 was a 6-week, Phase 3, randomized, placebo-controlled, efficacy study that enrolled 89 of the 96 responders from study PKU-001. PKU-003 demonstrated a statistically significant and consistent reduction in weekly blood Phe concentrations over 6 weeks with sapropterin (10 mg/kg/day) versus placebo (p<0.001) [13]. PKU-004, an open-label extension study to PKU-003, was a 22-week safety and efficacy Phase 3 study that enrolled 80 of the 87 subjects who completed PKU-003. PKU-004 showed that 5, 10, and 20 mg/kg/day doses were well-tolerated and led to sustained plasma Phe reductions over a 22-week period [14], and that once-daily dosing at ≥10 mg/kg can sustain stable blood Phe concentrations. In addition, this study demonstrated a dose-response relationship between sapropterin and blood Phe reduction. [14]. PKU-006, a two-part Phase 3 efficacy trial for sapropterin dosed at 20 mg/kg/day, was conducted on 90 PKU children aged 4–12 years with blood Phe concentrations under control with a Phe-restricted diet. Forty-six of the 50 sapropterin responders (defined as ≥30% decrease in blood Phe and blood Phe concentration ≤300 μmol/L) who were identified in the 8-day, open-label, Part 1 of PKU-006 enrolled in the 10-week, randomized, placebo-controlled, Part 2 of the study to assess tolerance to increased Phe intake. Children taking sapropterin had a significant reduction in blood Phe (p<0.001; Part 1) and a significant increase in Phe intake (p<0.001; Part 2) [15]. Both PKU-004 and PKU-006 trials demonstrated acceptable safety profiles, with no severe or serious treatment-related adverse events reported [14,15].

2. Materials and methods

This Phase 3b, multicenter, multinational, open-label study was a 3-year extension trial to evaluate the long-term safety of sapropterin in patients with PKU who participated in studies PKU-004 (after previously completing PKU-001 and PKU-003) or PKU-006. Subjects were enrolled at 15 sites in the United States and Canada and 13 European sites in the United Kingdom, France, Germany, Ireland, Italy, Poland, and Spain. Conduct of the protocol was approved at individual centers by local institutional review boards or ethics committees. Study PKU-008 began in July 2006. The study was conducted in accordance with the US Code of Federal Regulations for clinical research studies, the International Conference on Harmonization Guidelines for Good Clinical Practice, and the Declaration of Helsinki. The study was registered on ClinicalTrials.gov under the study registration number NCT00332189.

2.1. Subjects

Inclusion to PKU-008 was limited to sapropterin responders who completed either PKU-004 [14] or PKU-006 or subjects in PKU-006 who terminated early due to elevated Phe concentrations after experimental increases in Phe intake [15]. Exclusion criteria included a screening alanine aminotransferase value >2× upper limit of normal (ULN; Grade 1 or higher per WHO Toxicity Criteria); concurrent use of levodopa or folate inhibitors; and pregnant females or subjects of childbearing potential not currently using or unwilling to continue with birth control.

Informed written consent was obtained from all subjects before inclusion in the study. For children <18 years old, written informed consent was obtained from a parent or guardian, and children provided their assent, if required as per local regulations.

2.2. Study design

Fig. B.1 shows the series of PKU studies that led to enrollment in PKU-008. Some subjects were off of sapropterin therapy between completion of PKU-004 or PKU-006 and enrollment in PKU-008. After study PKU-008 was open for enrollment at their clinic site, subjects who were actively participating in studies PKU-004 or PKU-006 could enroll and participate in PKU-008 without interruption in therapy.

Subjects enrolled in PKU-008 were to receive once-daily oral administration of sapropterin and be evaluated for safety for up to three years (36 months) or until one of the following occurred: the subject withdrew consent and discontinued the study; the subject discontinued the study at the discretion of the investigator and in accordance with the investigator's clinical judgment; the drug became available via the appropriate marketing approval; or the study was terminated.

2.3. Dosing and mode of administration

Subjects were prescribed between 5 and 20 mg/kg/day oral sapropterin taken once daily and provided as tablets containing 100 mg of sapropterin each; daily doses were rounded up or down to the nearest 100 mg. All subjects who enrolled from PKU-004 began PKU-008 at the dose they were taking at the end of PKU-004. Because PKU-006 Part 2 was a blinded study and drug assignments were not revealed before subjects were enrolled in PKU-008, all subjects who enrolled from PKU-006 began PKU-008 at 20 mg/kg/day sapropterin despite PKU-006 treatment assignment (sapropterin or placebo). Investigators could adjust subjects' dose levels up or down in increments of approximately 5 mg/kg/day within a range of 5 to 20 mg/kg/day to control blood Phe concentrations in accordance with local clinical site recommendations.

Subjects dissolved sapropterin tablets in 4 to 8 oz (120 to 240 mL) of water or apple juice for at least the first 3 months. After a Phase 1 bioavailability study showed that taking intact tablets increased absorption by approximately 20% while maintaining an acceptable safety profile [16], the study was modified to allow dosing as intact tablets. Doses were to be taken before the morning meal. The study had no dietary restrictions. Phe intake was not monitored as part of this study; however, patients were advised to follow local site recommendations for dietary control and management of high blood Phe concentrations.

2.4. Study assessments

Safety was assessed by monitoring every 3 months for adverse events (AEs) and serious AEs (SAEs), clinical laboratory evaluations, physical examinations, concomitant medications, and vital sign measurements. Blood Phe concentrations were assessed 2.5 to 5 h after a meal. Abnormal test results determined to be clinically significant by the investigator, including results obtained at the final visit, were repeated until the cause of the abnormality was determined, the value returned to baseline or within normal limits, or the investigator determined that the abnormal value was no longer clinically significant.

2.5. Statistics

Safety analyses included subjects for whom post-dose safety data were available after taking at least one dose of study medication. Descriptive statistics were used to summarize the data. Categorical variables were summarized using frequencies and percentages.

Because this study was designed to monitor the safety of longer-term exposure to sapropterin, the study was neither randomized nor powered for efficacy. Consequently, there was no formal calculation for sample size. However, up to 128 subjects who participated in PKU-004 and PKU-006 Part 2 were eligible to enroll in PKU-008.

3. Results

3.1. Subject demographics and disposition

A total of 111 subjects enrolled in study PKU-008: 71 subjects were previously in study PKU-004, and 40 subjects were previously in PKU-006 (9 of these 40 subjects received placebo during study PKU-006) (Fig. B.1). Fifteen (7.4%) subjects transitioned from study PKU-004 or PKU-006 to study PKU-008 without interruption in treatment. For subjects transitioning from PKU-004, the mean duration of treatment interruption was 139 ± 86 days (range, 3–338 days). For subjects transitioning from PKU-006, the mean ± SD duration of treatment interruption (including placebo period for 9 subjects) was 76 ± 45 days (range, 15–122 days). Demographics of the study population are shown in Table A.1. The mean age of subjects enrolled in this study was 16.4 ± 10.2 years (range, 4 to 50 years). Approximately 65% of the population was <18 years old at the start of PKU-008. The distribution of age and race is consistent with the population characteristics of patients with PKU in North America and Europe [17]. One enrolled subject had an alanine aminotransferase value of 75 U/L that was considered not clinically significant but was higher than the 2× ULN exclusion cutoff. All other subjects met protocol inclusion requirements.

Subjects who enrolled in PKU-008 via participation in PKU-004 were considered completers if total exposure across all studies (PKU-001, PKU-003, PKU-004, and PKU-008) was ≥2 years; even after study drug became commercially available in the U.S., subjects in this group were allowed to continue in study PKU-008 until total exposure across all studies was 2 years. Subjects who enrolled in PKU-008 via participation in PKU-006 were considered completers when study drug became commercially available to the patient.

Twenty-one (18.9%) of the 111 subjects discontinued the study early. Three subjects discontinued because of an AE (one each of difficulty concentrating, clinically significant decreased platelet count, and intermittent diarrhea); all three events were considered possibly related to study drug treatment. Three subjects were withdrawn from the study at the Investigator's discretion due to uncooperative or noncompliant behavior. Nine subjects withdrew consent, four subjects were discontinued because the Investigator felt that the subject was unresponsive to sapropterin, and two subjects who moved out of country were withdrawn.

3.2. Exposure to study drug

The mean duration of exposure to sapropterin during PKU-008 was 658.7 ± 221.3 days (range, 56–953; median, 595 days). The maximum exposure to sapropterin during study PKU-008 was 953 days (2.6 years). Subjects who previously participated in PKU-001 (8 days), PKU-003 (42 days), and PKU-004 (154 days) had up to 204 days of exposure to sapropterin before enrollment to PKU-008. Subjects who previously participated in PKU-006 had up to 78 days of exposure to sapropterin before enrollment to PKU-008. The mean duration of exposure during participation in multiple studies (PKU-001, PKU-003, PKU-004, and PKU-008; or PKU-006 and PKU-008; see Fig. B.1) was 799.0 ± 237.5 days (range, 135-1151 days). The mean duration of exposure to sapropterin was 472.2 (±284.2) and 378.0 (±185.0) days when subjects were administered dissolved and intact tablets, respectively (subjects may have received both dissolved and intact tablets during total treatment duration).

Investigators could adjust subjects' dose levels up or down in increments of approximately 5 mg/kg/day. The median daily amount of sapropterin taken (prescribed dose divided by weight recorded at clinic visit) was 18.4 mg/kg/day (mean, 16.4 ± 4.4 mg/kg/day; range, 4.8–22.1 mg/kg/day). No difference in final mean dose of sapropterin was observed between subjects while taking intact tablets (16.8 ± 4.4 mg/kg/day) and dissolved tablets (16.2 ± 4.6 mg/kg/day). A lower percentage of subjects in the age range of 4–7 years took intact tablets, and subjects 4-7 years old had the highest final dose level (mean, 19.0 mg/kg/day; range, 15.2–20.7 mg/kg/day). Most deviations in compliance were considered minor and were not expected to affect safety analyses; overall, 94.6% of subjects were at least 80% compliant.

3.3. Safety

No new sapropterin-related safety signals were identified in this study. AEs were reported for 93 (83.8%) of the 111 subjects who received at least one dose of sapropterin. Drug-related AEs were reported for 37 (33.3%) of 111 subjects who received sapropterin. AEs were reported for 83 (75.5%) of 110 subjects while taking dissolved tablets and 44 (78.6%) of 56 subjects while taking intact tablets. Drug-related AEs were reported for 29 (26.4%) of 110 subjects while taking dissolved tablets and 11 (19.6%) of 56 subjects while taking intact tablets. Most AEs were considered to be mild or moderate. Of the severe AEs reported for six subjects, one subject had a severe AE that was considered to be possibly related to study drug treatment. The patient reported difficulty concentrating and mood swings. Timing of sapropterin treatment was altered so not to coincide with levothyroxin medication and the event resolved. Table A.2 lists AEs occurring in >5% of subjects. No drug-related AEs occurred at a frequency >5%. The most common drug-related AEs were viral gastroenteritis, vomiting, and headache (each 4.5% of subjects).

Three (2.7%) subjects withdrew from the study because of a drug-related AE (one each of difficulty concentrating, clinically significant decreased platelet count, and intermittent diarrhea). One subject with possible idiopathic thrombocytopenic purpura had consistently low platelet counts that were considered possibly related to study drug and resulted in study withdrawal (described in detail below). No other clinical laboratory results, vital sign measurements, or physical examinations revealed any clinically significant, drug-related AEs or changes. No age-related differences in AEs or other safety parameters were noted.

There were no deaths or discontinuations due to SAEs. Of the SAEs reported for seven subjects, one subject (while taking dissolved tablets) had an SAE that was considered to be probably related to study treatment. The patient was hospitalized for gastroesophageal reflux and the concomitant use of ibuprofen was identified as another possible cause for this event. Other SAEs included the report of a testicular mass and subsequent lymphadenectomy, incontinence requiring surgical correction, tonsillectomy, menorrhagia and dysmenorrhea, neck injury due to a traffic accident, and gastroesophageal reflux.

Of the subjects with baseline blood Phe levels within recommended reference ranges for PKU patients [3,18], most stayed within those reference ranges throughout the study. Approximately half of the subjects whose baseline blood Phe levels were considered above treatment guidelines shifted to within range during the study.

A blood Phe level ≤26 μmol/L was evaluated as a safety assessment because it was the lower limit of normal for healthy individuals 2 to 18 years old in the reference laboratory (Mayo Clinic, Department of Medical Laboratory and Pathology, Rochester, MN USA). Five (4.5%) subjects had seven occurrences of blood Phe levels ≤26 μmol/L. Twenty-seven (24%) subjects had blood Phe levels ≤120 μmol/L, which is the recommended lower limit for blood Phe in PKU patients [3,18]. These low blood Phe levels were transitory and were not associated with clinical symptoms. None of these events were reported as an AE or determined to be clinically significant, and all resolved without intervention.

There were no clinically relevant mean changes over time for any hematology or clinical chemistry parameter, including liver function tests. Two subjects had clinically significant ALT and AST values. For one subject, clinically significant ALT and AST values were reported at 15 months; ALT and AST levels then decreased through early termination 2 months later (subject withdrew consent), at which time AST had normalized and ALT had decreased to a high but clinically insignificant level. For the second subject, clinically significant ALT and AST values were reported at 3 months; ALT levels dropped to a high but clinically insignificant level and AST levels were still high and clinically significant at early termination 1 month later (subject withdrew consent). Both ALT and AST levels were normal 1 month after termination.

Neutropenia has been reported in previous sapropterin studies [14,15]. In study PKU-008, neutrophil counts <1.0×10^9/L were reported for three subjects at one timepoint each. Twenty-one other subjects had neutrophil counts between 1.0 and 1.5×10^9/L at one or more timepoints. Altogether, 24 subjects had neutrophil counts <1.5×10^9/L at 35 timepoints. All decreases in neutrophil counts were transitory and did not require intervention. There were no significant decreases in other hematopoietic lineages (ie, platelets and red blood cells) correlating with decreased neutrophil counts, and neutrophil counts did not trend downward during participation in PKU-008.

Thirteen subjects had one or more platelet counts below the lower limit of normal. Generally these subjects had low-normal (150 to 200×10^9/L) to low (<150×10^9/L) platelet counts at baseline, and changes did not appear to be associated with study drug exposure. Four of these 13 subjects had one or more platelet counts below 100×10^9/L. One subject who had low platelet counts before any exposure to study drug (98×10^9/L at PKU-001 screening) and through participation in studies PKU-001, PKU-003, and PKU-004 continued to have low platelet counts during participation in PKU-008 (below 100×10^9/L, including a baseline count of 77×10^9/L). At the Month 15 visit, the platelet count was considered clinically significant at 37×10^9/L. The subject was withdrawn from the study 2 months later (65×10^9/L at withdrawal). This subject's thrombocytopenia was considered by the Investigator to be related to idiopathic thrombocytopenic purpura. This AE was ongoing at the end of the study, and the subject was referred to a hematologist. No follow-up information is available.

4. Discussion

These data represent the longest exposure to sapropterin in controlled clinical trials, with subjects receiving up to 2.6 years of sapropterin treatment. Study PKU-008 had a safety profile that was consistent with previous studies on which regulatory approval of sapropterin was based and for which PKU-008 was an extension (PKU-001, PKU-003, PKU-004, and PKU-006 [12–15]).

The majority of subjects who began treatment at 10 mg/kg/day were eventually prescribed 20 mg/kg/day of sapropterin, which was administered as both dissolved and intact tablets during this study. A lower percentage of children in the 4- to 7-year-old age group transitioned to intact tablets, likely because children in this age range can have difficulty swallowing intact tablets. There were no notable differences in the incidence and severity of AEs when sapropterin was administered as a dissolved or intact tablet. Because duration of exposure was longer for dissolved compared to intact tablets and fewer younger children transitioned to intact tablets, a direct comparison between the rates of AEs between the two dosing regimens cannot be made.

Overall, AEs reported for subjects treated with sapropterin were consistent with those seen in other studies [13–15]. The proportion of subjects experiencing an AE (84%) was similar to safety reports of the PKU-004 (85%) and PKU-006 (76%) studies, and most AEs reported in PKU-008 were mild and considered unrelated to study drug. Severe AEs were reported in six subjects of which only one was related to study drug while no drug related severe AEs were reported in the PKU-004 [14] and PKU-006 [15] studies. The most common AEs (>5% of subjects) observed in the current study that were consistent with previous studies included headache, rhinorrhea, pharyngolaryngeal pain, diarrhea, and vomiting.

Overall, the SAE profile was similar to the results of the PKU-004 and PKU-006 studies. There were no deaths or discontinuations from the study due to SAEs. There were seven SAEs reported in the current study, however only one SAE was related to study drug. This compares well with one study drug related SAE in PKU-004 [14] and no study drug related SAEs in PKU-006 [15].

While data were not analyzed based on age populations in PKU-008, the occurrence of treatment related severe AEs and SAEs in the long term follow-up of subjects in the PKU-008 study remained similar to those of patients 4–12 years old (PKU-006) [15] and patients ≥8 years old (PKU-004) [14]. In addition, there does not appear to be an increased risk at higher dose levels of sapropterin up to 20 mg/kg/day The AE profiles observed in PKU-004, PKU-006 and PKU-008 are at dose levels equivalent to, or greater than those recommended in previous published studies (2–10 mg/kg/day) for treatment of tetrahydrobiopterin (BH_4) deficiency in children and adults [18,19].

The range of blood Phe levels considered optimal for patients with PKU varies among healthcare professionals, and guidelines differ from country to country [3,20–23]. For the purpose of this study, 26 μmol/L (the lower limit of age-related normal Phe level at the Department of Medical Laboratory and Pathology), and 120 μmol/L (the lower limit that should be targeted in PKU patients [3,20]) were used to define low blood Phe levels. Blood Phe levels fell below what was considered the lower limits only sporadically. In PKU-008, 5 (4.5%) subjects treated with 5–20 mg/kg/day sapropterin, were reported to have had a Phe level <26 μmol/L. In contrast, 13 of 33 (39%) patients in the PKU-006 study reached a blood Phe <26 μmol/L at a fixed dose of 20 mg/kg/day and blood Phe levels subsequently increased in all subject to ≥26 μmol/L when the diet was modified to increase Phe intake. In both studies, the low blood Phe levels were transient and were not associated with any AEs. None of the occurrences of blood Phe <26 μmol/L were determined to be clinically significant and all resolved without intervention. It is clear that low blood Phe levels may occur in PKU patients during sapropterin treatment or if dietary Phe intake is too restricted; therefore, treatment with sapropterin should be monitored and dietary Phe intake adjusted based on blood Phe levels and management of the individual patient.

Although efficacy outcomes were not specifically addressed in this long-term extension study, controlled blood Phe levels throughout the study confirm the durability of response in subjects of all ages who are undergoing long-term treatment with sapropterin and who were previously either adhering (PKU-006) or not adhering (PKU-004) to diet.

5. Conclusion

In this study, sapropterin was found to be safe and well-tolerated at doses of 5 to 20 mg/kg/day for up to 2.6 years while controlling blood Phe levels. This study supports the safety and tolerability of sapropterin as long-term treatment for patients with PKU.

Potential conflicts of interest

BK Burton and DK Grange have received grant support, honoraria, and consulting fees from BioMarin Pharmaceutical, Inc. A. Dorenbaum is a former employee and current shareholder of BioMarin Pharmaceutical, Inc. M. Imperiale and S. Kim are current employees and shareholders of BioMarin Pharmaceutical, Inc.

Submission declaration

The work described herein has not been published previously except as an abstract (Fernhoff PM, Burton BK, Nowacka M, Hennermann JB, Kakkis E, Dorenbaum A. PKU-008: a long-term, open-label study of sapropterin dihydrochloride [Kuvan®] in PKU subjects. American College of Medical Genetics [ACMG] Annual Meeting. Tampa, FL, March 25–29, 2009. Abstract 190.), is not under consideration for publication elsewhere, and has been approved by all authors as well as the authorities where the work was conducted. If accepted, these data will not be published elsewhere, including electronically in the same form, in English or any other language, without the written consent of the copyright holder.

Source of funding

This study was sponsored by BioMarin Pharmaceutical, Inc.

Study registration number

NCT00332189 (http://ClinicalTrials.gov).

Acknowledgments

The authors thank their fellow investigators of the Sapropterin Research Group: Stephen Cederbaum, UCLA Medical Center, Los Angeles, CA, USA; Lorne Clarke, University of British Columbia, Vancouver, BC, Canada; Maureen Cleary, Great Ormond Street Hospital, London, UK; Dries Dobbelaere, Hôpital Jeanne de Flandres, Lille, France; Annette Feigenbaum, Hospital for Sick Children, Toronto, ON, Canada; Francois Feillet, Hôpital d'Enfants, Vandoeuvre les Nancy, France; Marcello Giovannini, Azienda Ospedaliera San Paolo, Milan, Italy; Cary Harding, Oregon Health & Science University, Portland, OR, USA; Philip Lee, National Hospital for Neurology and Neurosurgery, London, UK; Nicola Longo, University of Utah, Salt Lake City, UT, USA; Mercedes Martinez-Pardo Casanova, Hospital Ramón y Cajal, Madrid, Spain; Concetta Meli, Azienda Ospedaliera Universitaria, Catania, Italy; Andrew Morris, Royal Manchester Children's Hospital, Manchester, UK; Linda Randolph, Children's Hospital Los Angeles, Los Angeles, CA, USA; Margretta Seashore, Yale University School of Medicine, New Haven, CT, USA; Eileen P. Treacy, The Children's University Hospital, Dublin, Ireland; Lewis Waber, University of Texas Southwestern Medical Center, Dallas, TX, USA; Melissa Wasserstein, Mount Sinai Medical Center, New York, NY, USA; Chester B. Whitley, University of Minnesota, Minneapolis, MN, USA; and Jon Wolff, University of Wisconsin, Madison, WI, USA.

Becky Stein Norquist and Curtis Gravance provided medical writing services and Bae Cheng and Chris Barker provided statistical analysis services on behalf of BioMarin Pharmaceutical, Inc.

Appendix A. Tables

Table A.1
Summary characteristics of the PKU-008 study population.

Characteristic	Study population
Age range, years	
Mean ± SD (range)	16.4 ± 10.2 (4–50)
≥ 4 to < 8, n (%)	20 (18.0)
≥ 8 to < 12, n (%)	24 (21.6)
≥ 12 to < 18, n (%)	28 (25.2)
≥ 18, n (%)	39 (35.1)
Sex	
Male, n (%)	67 (60.4)
Female, n (%)	44 (39.6)
Race	
White, n (%)	108 (97.3)
Other, n (%)[a]	3 (2.7)
Clinical site location	
North America, n (%)	54 (48.6)
Europe, n (%)	57 (51.4)
Enrolled from preceding clinical trial	
PKU-004, n (%)	71 (64.0)
PKU-006, n (%)	40 (36.0)
Baseline blood Phe level (μmol/L) at Day 0 of study[b]	
PKU-004, mean ± SD (range)	769.2 ± 396.2 (53–1573)
PKU-006, mean ± SD (range)	317.0 ± 173.2 (49–824)
PKU-008, mean ± SD (range)	613.1 ± 328.5 (10–1533)

[a] Other race includes Asian, Hispanic, and Other categories, which had one subject each.
[b] Nine subjects from study PKU-006 were in the placebo group before enrolling in study PKU-008. Most subjects had a discontinuation of sapropterin treatment between completion of study PKU-004 or PKU-006 and initiation of sapropterin treatment in PKU-008.

Table A.2
Treatment-emergent adverse events and drug-related treatment-emergent adverse events occurring in >5% of subjects.

System organ class Preferred term	No. of subjects (%), no. of events									
	All TEAEs[a]					Drug-related TEAEs[b]				
	4–7 years (N=20)	8–11 years (N=24)	12–17 years (N=28)	≥18 years (N=39)	Total (N=111)	4–7 years (N=20)	8–11 years (N=24)	12–17 years (N=28)	≥18 years (N=39)	Total (N=111)
Infection and infestations	20 (100), 58	17 (70.8), 42	14 (50.0), 32	23 (59.0), 66	74 (66.7), 198	3 (15.0), 8	2 (8.3), 4	3 (10.7), 1	3 (7.7), 5	11 (9.9), 27
Upper respiratory tract infection	6 (30.0), 10	7 (29.2), 7	6 (21.4), 7	3 (7.7), 4	22 (19.8), 28	0	0	2 (7.1), 2	0	2 (1.8), 2
Nasopharyngitis	2 (10.0), 4	1 (4.2), 1	5 (17.9), 8	12 (30.8), 17	20 (18.0), 30	0	0	2 (7.1), 5	1 (2.6), 1	3 (2.7), 6
Influenza	3 (15.0), 5	1 (4.2), 1	1 (3.6), 1	4 (10.3), 8	9 (8.1), 15	0	0	0	1 (2.6), 2	1 (0.9), 2
Viral infection	5 (25.0), 8	1 (4.2), 2	1 (3.6), 1	1 (2.6), 1	8 (7.2), 12	1 (5.0), 1	0	0	0	1 (0.9), 1
Gastroenteritis viral	2 (10.0), 2	3 (12.5), 4	2 (7.1), 2	1 (2.6), 1	8 (7.2), 9	2 (10.0), 2	1 (4.2), 2	2 (7.1), 2	0	5 (4.5), 6
Pharyngitis	1 (5.0), 1	4 (16.7), 10	0	2 (5.1), 2	7 (6.3), 13	0	0	0	0	0
Gastroenteritis	2 (10.0), 2	1 (4.2), 1	2 (7.1), 2	2 (5.1), 2	7 (6.3), 7	0	0	0	0	0
Bronchitis	2 (10.0), 2	1 (4.2), 1	0	3 (7.7), 4	6 (5.4), 7	0	0	0	0	0
Gastrointestinal disorders	11 (55.0), 16	9 (37.5), 16	8 (28.6), 12	15 (38.5), 29	43 (38.7), 73	4 (20.0), 5	0	4 (14.3), 5	6 (15.4), 8	14 (12.6), 18
Vomiting	6 (30.0), 6	5 (20.8), 6	4 (14.3), 5	5 (12.8), 7	20 (18.0), 24	3 (15.0), 3	0	0	2 (5.1), 3	5 (4.5), 6
Diarrhea	1 (5.0), 1	3 (12.5), 6	1 (3.6), 1	5 (12.8), 8	10 (9.0), 16	0	0	1 (3.6), 1	2 (5.1), 2	3 (2.7), 3
Respiratory, thoracic, and midiastinal disorders	7 (35.0), 18	9 (37.5), 26	8 (28.6), 17	12 (30.8), 16	36 (32.4), 77	1 (5.0), 2	2 (8.3), 6	0	1 (2.6), 1	4 (3.6), 9
Cough	4 (20.0), 8	6 (25.0), 8	4 (14.3), 5	7 (17.9), 7	21 (18.9), 28	1 (5.0), 2	1 (4.2), 2	0	1 (2.6), 1	3 (2.7), 5
Pharyngolaryngeal pain	0	6 (25.0), 11	2 (7.1), 2	2 (5.1), 2	10 (9.0), 15	0	1 (4.2), 4	0	0	1 (0.9), 4
Nasal congestion	2 (10.0), 2	2 (8.3), 4	3 (10.7), 5	2 (5.1), 2	9 (8.1), 13	0	0	0	0	0
Rhinorrhoea	3 (15.0), 4	1 (4.2), 2	2 (7.1), 2	0	6 (5.4), 8	0	0	0	0	0
General disorders and administration site conditions	8 (40.0), 9	6 (25.0), 12	5 (17.9), 6	6 (15.4), 6	25 (22.5), 33	2 (10.0), 2	2 (8.3), 3	0	0	4 (3.6), 5
Pyrexia	8 (40.0), 9	5 (20.8), 3	3 (10.7), 4	2 (5.1), 2	18 (16.2), 25	2 (10.0), 2	2 (8.3), 3	0	0	4 (3.6), 5
Nervous system disorders	2 (10.0), 3	4 (16.7), 7	4 (14.3), 8	6 (15.4), 35	16 (14.4), 53	1 (5.0), 1	0	0	5 (12.8), 24	6 (5.4), 25
Headache	2 (10.0), 3	3 (12.5), 6	3 (10.7), 7	5 (12.8), 32	13 (11.7), 48	1 (5.0), 1	0	0	4 (10.3), 22	5 (4.5), 23

TEAE: treatment-emergent adverse event.
The three values in each column represent the number of subjects (%) who reported an event and the frequency of the AE.
[a] The total number of TEAEs may be greater than the total number subjects because subjects may have experienced more than one adverse event.
[b] Related adverse events include adverse events that were considered possibly or probably related to study drug.

Appendix B. Figures

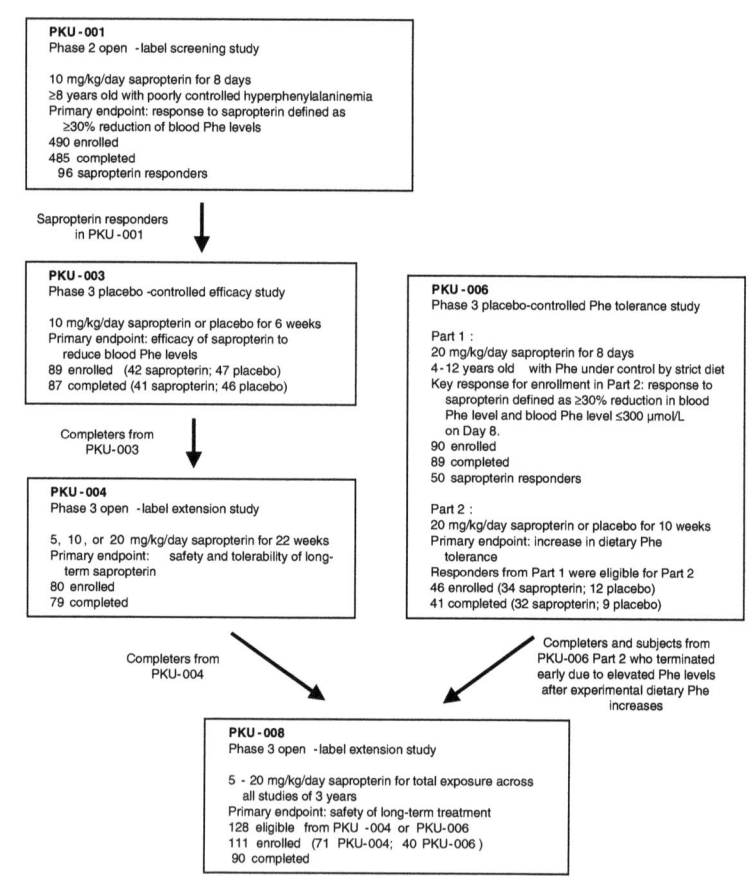

Fig. B.1. Subject flow through clinical trials.

References

[1] C.R. Scriver, S. Kaufman, Hyperphenylalaninemia: phenylalanine hydroxylase deficiency, in: A.L. Beaudet, W.S. Sly, D. Valle (Eds.), Metabolic and Molecular Bases of Inherited Disease, McGraw-Hill, New York, 2001, pp. 1667–1709.
[2] J.J. Moyle, A.M. Fox, M. Arthur, M. Bynevelt, J.R. Burnett, Meta-analysis of neuropsychological symptoms of adolescents and adults with PKU, Neuropsychol. Rev. 17 (2007) 91–101.
[3] National Institutes of Health, Phenylketonuria (PKU): screening and management, NIH Consens. Statement 17 (3) (2000) 1–33.
[4] A. MacDonald, H. Gokmen-Ozel, M. van Rijn, P. Burgard, The reality of dietary compliance in the management of phenylketonuria, J. Inherit. Metab. Dis. 33 (6) (2010) 665–670.
[5] S. Kure, D.C. Hou, T. Ohura, H. Iwamoto, S. Suzuki, N. Sugiyama, O. Sakamoto, K. Fujii, Y. Matsubara, K. Narisawa, Tetrahydrobiopterin-responsive phenylalanine hydroxylase deficiency, J. Pediatr. 135 (1999) 375–378.
[6] A.C. Muntau, W. Roschinger, M. Habich, H. Demmelmair, B. Hoffmann, C.P. Sommerhoff, A.A. Roscher, Tetrahydrobiopterin as an alternative treatment for mild phenylketonuria, N. Engl. J. Med. 347 (2002) 2122–2132.
[7] H. Shintaku, S. Kure, T. Ohura, Y. Okano, M. Ohwada, N. Sugiyama, N. Sakura, I. Yoshida, M. Yoshino, Y. Matsubara, K. Suzuki, K. Aoki, T. Kitagawa, Long-term treatment and diagnosis of tetrahydrobiopterin-responsive hyperphenylalaninemia with a mutant phenylalanine hydroxylase gene, Pediatr. Res. 55 (2004) 425–430.
[8] F.K. Trefz, C. Aulela-Scholz, N. Blau, Successful treatment of phenylketonuria with tetrahydrobiopterin, Eur. J. Pediatr. 160 (2001) 315.
[9] R. Steinfeld, A. Kohlschutter, K. Ullrich, Z. Lukacs, Efficiency of long-term tetrahydrobiopterin monotherapy in phenylketonuria, J. Inherit. Metab. Dis. 27 (2004) 449–453.
[10] J.B. Hennermann, C. Buhrer, N. Blau, B. Vetter, E. Monch, Long-term treatment with tetrahydrobiopterin increases phenylalanine tolerance in children with severe phenotype of phenylketonuria, Mol. Genet. Metab. 86 (Suppl. 1) (2005) S86–S90.

[11] M.J. Belanger-Quintana, M. Garcia, L.R. Castro, B. Desviat, B. Perez, M. Mejia, M. Ugarte, M. Martinez-Pardo, Spanish BH$_4$-responsive phenylalanine hydroxylase-deficient patients: evolution of seven patients on long-term treatment with tetrahydrobiopterin, Mol. Genet. Metab. 86 (Suppl. 1) (2005) S61–S66.
[12] B.K. Burton, D.K. Grange, A. Milanowski, G. Vockley, F. Feillet, E.A. Crombez, V. Abadie, C.O. Harding, S. Cederbaum, D. Dobbelaere, A. Smith, A. Dorenbaum, The response of patients with phenylketonuria and elevated serum phenylalanine to treatment with oral sapropterin dihydrochloride (6R-tetrahydrobiopterin): a Phase II, multicentre, open-label, screening study, J. Inherit. Metab. Dis. 30 (2007) 700–707.
[13] H. Levy, A. Milanowski, A. Chakrapani, M. Cleary, P. Lee, F.K. Trefz, C.B. Whitley, F. Feillet, A.S. Feigenbaum, J. Bebchuk, H. Christ-Schmidt, A. Dorenbaum, Sapropterin Research Group, Efficacy of sapropterin dihydrochloride (tetrahydrobiopterin, 6R-BH$_4$) for reduction of phenylalanine concentration in patients with phenylketonuria: a Phase III randomized placebo-controlled study, Lancet 370 (2007) 504–510.
[14] P. Lee, E.P. Treacy, E. Crombez, M. Wasserstein, L. Waber, J. Wolff, U. Wendel, A. Dorenbaum, J. Bebchuk, H. Christ-Schmidt, M. Seashore, M. Giovannini, B.K. Burton, A.A. Morris, the Sapropterin Research Group, Safety and efficacy of 22 weeks of treatment with sapropterin dihydrochloride in patients with phenylketonuria, Am. J. Med. Genet. A 146A (2008) 2851–2859.
[15] F.K. Trefz, B.K. Burton, N. Longo, M.M. Casanova, D.J. Gruskin, A. Dorenbaum, E.D. Kakkis, E.A. Crombez, D.K. Grange, P. Harmatz, M.H. Lipson, A. Milanowski, L.M. Randolph, J. Vockley, C.B. Whitley, J.A. Wolff, J. Bebchuk, H. Christ-Schmidt, J.B. Hennermann, for the Sapropterin Study Group, Efficacy of sapropterin dihydrochloride in increasing phenylalanine tolerance in children with phenylketonuria: a Phase III, randomized, double-blind, placebo-controlled study, J. Pediatr. 154 (2009) 700–707.
[16] D. Musson, C. O'Neill, W. Kramer, E. Foehr, P. Bieberdorf, S. Kim, A. Dorenbaum, S. Turbeville, H. Nicely, The bioavailability of Kuvan™ (sapropterin dihydrochloride) from intact or dissolved tablets administered with or without food to healthy volunteers, Poster Presentation at 2007 Meeting of the Society for Inherited Metabolic Disorders, March 2007, Asilomar, CA.
[17] Z.P. Mijuskovic, D. Karadaglic, L. Stajanov, Phenylketonuria, Available at: emedicine.medscape.com/article/1115450-overview, Accessed 18 August 2010.
[18] L. Jaggi, M.R. Zurfluh, A. Schuler, A. Ponzone, P. Francesco, L. Fiori, M. Giovannini, R. Santer, G.F. Hoffmann, H. Ibel, U. Wendel, D. Ballhausen, M.R. Baumgartner, N. Blau, Outcome and long-term follow-up of 36 patients with tetrahydrobiopterin deficiency, Mol. Genet. Metab. 93 (2008) 295–305.
[19] N. Blau, G.F. Hoffman, J. Leonard, J.T.R. Clarke (Eds.), Physician's Guide to the Treatment and Follow-up of Metabolic Diseases, Springer, Berlin, 2006, pp. 25–34.
[20] Medical Research Council Working Party on Phenylketonuria, Recommendations on the dietary management of phenylketonuria, Arch. Dis. Child. 68 (1993) 426–427.
[21] J. Bekhof, M. van Rijn, P.J.J. Sauer, E.M. Ten Vergert, D.-J. Reijngoud, F.J. van Spronsen, Plasma phenylalanine in patients with phenylketonuria self-managing their diet, Arch. Dis. Child. 90 (2005) 163–164.
[22] P. Burgard, H.J. Bremer, P. Bührdel, P.C. Clemens, E. Mönch, H. Przyrembel, F.K. Trefz, K. Ullrich, Rationale for the German recommendations for phenylalanine level control in phenylketonuria 1997, Eur. J. Pediatr. 158 (1999) 46–54.
[23] V. Abadie, J. Berthelot, F. Feillet, N. Maurin, A. Mercier, H. Ogier de Baulny, L. de Parscau, Management of phenylketonuria and hyperphenylalaninemia: the French guidelines [article in French], Arch. Pediatr. 12 (2005) 594–601.

2.6. PUBLIKATION 6: **Hennermann JB**, Roloff S, Gebauer C, Vetter B, von Arnim-Baas A, Mönch E. Long-term treatment with tetrahydrobiopterin in phenylketonuria: Treatment strategies and prediction of long-term responders. 2012. Mol Genet Metab 107:294-301. DOI 10.1016/j.ymgme.2012.09.021

Reprinted from: Molecular Genetics and Metabolism 2012, Volume 107 (3), page 294-301, with permission from Elsevier Inc., 2012, provided by Copyright Clearance Center

Trotz der Erstbeschreibung der BH4-responsiven PKU vor mehr als 10 Jahren fehlen weiterhin Empfehlungen zur Identifizierung von PKU-Patienten, die langzeit-BH4-responsiv sind. Ziel dieser Studie war daher zum einen die Identifizierung von Parametern, die eine Langzeit-BH4-Responsivität vorhersagen, zum anderen die Etablierung eines strukturierten Prozederes zur Etablierung der BH4-Langzeittherapie.

Wir untersuchten 116 diätpflichtige PKU-Patienten im Alter von 4-18 Jahren (Median 8,8 Jahre) auf ihre mögliche Langzeit-BH4-Responsivität. Patienten mussten mindestens zwei der folgenden drei Kriterien erfüllen: positiver neonataler BH4-Belastungstest, potentiell BH4-responsiver Genotyp, milder Phänotyp. 23/116 Patienten erfüllten die Einschlusskriterien und erhielten eine BH4-Langzeittherapie über mindestens drei Monate. Die Steigerung der diätetischen Phe-Zufuhr sowie die Anpassung der Aminosäuren-Zufuhr erfolgten nach einem genau definierten Protokoll. Die Therapie mit BH4 wurde bei allen Patienten in einer Dosierung von 20 mg/kg KG/Tag gestartet und nach Protokoll reduziert. Änderungen der Diät sowie der BH4-Gabe erfolgten abhängig von den jeweiligen Phe-Plasmakonzentrationen.

18 der 23 selektierten Patienten zeigten ein dauerhaftes Ansprechen auf die Behandlung mit BH4, 5 dagegen nicht. Die 18 Patienten, die dauerhaft auf die Therapie mit BH4 ansprachen, wurden über einen Zeitraum von 48 ± 27 Monaten mit einer BH4-Dosis von 14,9 ± 3,3 mg/kg KG/Tag behandelt. Unter der BH4-Therapie konnte die initiale Phe-Toleranz von 452 ± 201 mg/Tag auf 1593 ± 647 mg/Tag gesteigert werden, was einem Anstieg der Phe-Toleranz um 275 ± 151% entsprach. Bei 8 der 18 mit BH4 behandelten Patienten konnte das Phe-freie Aminosäurengemisch abgesetzt werden, 10 Patienten benötigten weiterhin ein Aminosäurengemisch in einer Dosierung von 0,63 ± 0,23 g Protein/kg KG/Tag. 7/18 Patienten berichteten über gastrointestinale Nebenwirkungen unter der BH4-Therapie.

Wir verglichen die laborchemischen, klinischen und molekulargenetischen Daten der Patienten, die langzeit-BH4-responsiv waren, mit denen der Patienten, die nicht langzeit-BH4-responsiv waren. Die Kombination folgender Parameter ergab den höchsten prädiktiven Wert für Langzeit-BH4-Responsivität: Phe-Konzentration bei Diagnosestellung <1200 µmol/L, Phe/Tyr-Ratio bei Diagnosestellung <15, Phe/Tyr-Ratio unter diätetischer Behandlung <15, Phe-Toleranz im Alter von drei Jahren >20 mg/kg KG/Tag, positiver neonataler BH4-Belastungstest und mindestens eine potentiell BH4-responsive Mutation (p = 0,00024). Sogar bei Vergleich der Parameter, die bereits kurz nach Diagnosestellung in der Neonatalperiode verfügbar sind (Phe-Konzentration und Phe/Tyr-Ratio bei Diagnosestellung, neonataler BH4-Belastungstest und Genotyp), ergab sich ein signifikanter Unterschied zwischen der Gruppe der Langzeit-BH4-Responder und der Nicht-Responder (p = 0,02).

Anhand der in dieser Studie identifizierten Parameter wird es möglich, bereits kurz nach der Diagnosestellung einer PKU eine potentielle Langzeit-BH4-Responsivität vorherzusagen und somit früh die Entscheidung über eine eventuelle BH4-Therapie zu treffen.

Long-term treatment with tetrahydrobiopterin in phenylketonuria: Treatment strategies and prediction of long-term responders

Julia B. Hennermann, Sylvia Roloff, Christine Gebauer, Barbara Vetter, Annabel von Arnim-Baas, Eberhard Mönch

Otto Heubner Center for Pediatric and Adolescent Medicine, Charité Universitätsmedizin Berlin, Germany

article info

Article history:
Received 11 August 2012
Received in revised form 21 September 2012
Accepted 21 September 2012
Available online 27 September 2012

Keywords:
Hyperphenylalaninemia
Phenylketonuria
Tetrahydrobiopterin
Sapropterin

abstract

Tetrahydrobiopterin (BH4) responsive phenylketonuria has been described more than 10 years ago. However, criteria for the identification of long-term BH4 responsive patients are not yet established. 116 patients with phenylketonuria, aged 4–18 years, were screened for potential long-term BH4 responsiveness by at least two of the following criteria: positive neonatal BH4 loading test, putative BH4 responsive genotype, and/or milder phenotype. Patients had to be on permanent dietary treatment. 23 patients fulfilled these criteria and were tested for long-term BH4 responsiveness: 18/23 were long-term BH4 responsive, 5/23 were not.

On long-term BH4 treatment over a period of 48±27 months in a dose of 14.9±3.3 mg/kg/day phenylalanine tolerance was increased from 452±201 mg/day to 1593±647 mg/day, corresponding to a mean increase of 1141±528 mg/day. Dietary phenylalanine intake was increased stepwise according to a clear defined protocol. In 8/18 patients, diet was completely liberalized; 10/18 patients still received phenylalanine-free amino acid formula with 0.63±0.23 g/kg/day.

The most predictive value for long-term BH4 responsiveness was the combination of pretreatment phenylalanine of ≤1200 μmol/L, pretreatment phenylalanine/tyrosine ratio of ≤15, phenylalanine/tyrosine ratio of ≤15 on treatment, phenylalanine tolerance of >20 mg/kg/day at age 3 years, positive neonatal BH4 loading, and at least one putative BH4 responsive mutation (p=0.00024).

Our data show that long-term BH4 responsiveness may be predicted already during neonatal period by determining maximum pretreatment phenylalanine and phenylalanine/tyrosine concentrations, neonatal BH4 loading, and *PAH* genotype. A clear defined protocol is necessary to install long-term BH4 treatment.

© 2012 Elsevier Inc. All rights reserved.

1. Introduction

Phenylketonuria (PKU, MIM 261600) is a rare autosomal recessive inborn error of metabolism caused by phenylalanine-4-hydroxylase (PAH, EC 1.14.16.1) deficiency [1]. In untreated children, PKU results in severe neurological impairment with mental retardation, seizures, and behavioral disorders. Normal mental and motor activity skills can be achieved by early institution of a phenylalanine (Phe)-restricted diet consisting of a strong restriction of natural protein intake and substitution with a Phe-free L-amino acid formula [1]. Dietary treatment has been improved over the past decades, by improving taste and composition of amino acid mixtures and by introducing special low protein food products. However, compliance to Phe-restricted diet is challenging and decreases with age, mainly during puberty and adolescence. Within the last decade, new therapeutic approaches for patients with PKU have been established. In 1999, the treatment of PKU patients with tetrahydrobiopterin (BH4), the cofactor of PAH, has been described for the first time [2]. Since then, multiple studies reported on the effect of BH4 in PKU patients with PAH deficiency [3–11].

The introduction of BH4 has been regarded with growing enthusiasm and optimism. It has been estimated that at least 30–40% of the PKU patients may benefit from BH4 treatment [12,13]. However, most studies on BH4 treatment in PKU patients have only been performed over a short period of time; and few studies only examine the long-term effect of BH4 treatment. Additionally, the majority of studies on BH4 treatment emphasize on the effect of decreasing Phe levels [4,5,14], and only a few on the effect of increasing Phe tolerance. These studies reported a two- to three-fold increase in individual Phe tolerance on BH4 treatment [8–10]. However, in the day-to-day care of patients, the increase in Phe tolerance is more relevant, as liberalization of the diet is associated with an improvement of the patients' adherence to treatment and their quality of life. Recently, North American recommendations for the use of BH4 have

---

Abbreviations: BH4, tetrahydrobiopterin; HPA, hyperphenylalaninemia; PAH, phenylalanine hydroxylase; Phe, phenylalanine; PKU, phenylketonuria; Tyr, tyrosine.
⁎ Corresponding author at: Otto Heubner Center for Pediatric and Adolescent Medicine, Department of Pediatric Endocrinology, Gastroenterology and Metabolic Diseases, Charité Universitätsmedizin Berlin, Augustenburger Platz 1, 13353 Berlin, Germany. Fax: +49 30 450566918.
E-mail address: julia.hennermann@charite.de (J.B. Hennermann).

1096-7192/$ – see front matter © 2012 Elsevier Inc. All rights reserved.
http://dx.doi.org/10.1016/j.ymgme.2012.09.021

been established [15]. However, the identi cation of PKU patients, who may bene t from a long-term treatment with BH4, still remains challenging.

In this study, we emphasize the effect of long-term BH4 treatment on increasing the individual Phe tolerance. We developed an effective approach for implementing long-term BH4 treatment with individual increases of dietary Phe intake and individual dosing of BH4. Furthermore, we identi ed parameters which may help to early predict long-term BH4 responsiveness in patients with PKU.

2. Patients and methods

2.1. Patients

116 patients with PKU, aged 4–18 years (median age 8.8 years), treated in the metabolic unit of the Department of Pediatrics at the Charité Berlin were examined for their potential BH4-responsiveness. 114/116 patients were diagnosed by newborn screening within the rst two weeks of life; two patients, not born in Germany, were diagnosed by selective screening at the age of 6 and 18 months, respectively. Neonatal BH4 loading test was performed in all patients with an initial Phe plasma value of ≥ 400 mol/L (84/114). In 56 patients, neonatal BH4 loading test was performed over a period of 24 h, in 26 patients over a period of 8 h. In two patients, who had initially been treated in another center, results of neonatal BH4 test were not available. BH4 loading test was classi ed as positive when Phe value decreased ≥ 30% from baseline. According to established criteria [16–18], 44% of the patients were classi ed as classic PKU (n = 51), 15.5% as mild PKU (n = 18) and 40.5% as hyperphenylalaninemia (HPA) (n = 47).

Patients were screened for potential long-term BH4 responsiveness by proof of at least two of the following criteria: a mild PKU phenotype, a positive neonatal BH4 loading test, and/or at least one potential BH4 responsive mutation. Exclusion criteria were patients with poor compliance to treatment, patients with HPA who did not receive any treatment, pregnancy, and refusal of BH4 treatment. According to the German recommendations for treatment in PKU [19], only patients with Phe plasma concentrations of >600 mol/L received treatment. All parents gave informed consent to BH4 treatment and data analyses.

2.2. Definition of long-term BH4 responsiveness

Primary goal of long-term BH4 treatment was a signi cant increase in Phe tolerance while maintaining a good metabolic control. A signi cant increase in Phe tolerance was de ned as an increase in Phe tolerance to at least 2.5-fold, corresponding to previous studies reporting a 2- to 3-fold increase in Phe tolerance on BH4 treatment [8–10]. BH4 treatment was discontinued, if Phe increase was b 2.0-fold after a period of 3 months and b 2.5-fold after a period of 4 months, if Phe plasma levels increased above the recommended levels, according to age and according to the German recommendations for the treatment in PKU [19], and/or if patients were incompliant to BH4 treatment. Secondary goals were an increase in quality of life, a continuous stabilization of metabolic control, and an optimal supply with protein, vitamins and micronutrients.

2.3. Control of diet and modification of diet on long-term BH4 treatment

Optimal compliance and cooperation of the patients and their parents was required to start long-term BH4 treatment. Patients were examined every 3 months in our metabolic unit, including height and weight. Dietary protocols were calculated every 6 months, with focus on the intake of protein, calories, vitamins and micronutrients.

On BH4 treatment, Phe intake was increased weekly if Phe levels were within the recommended range according to the patient's age and the patient's individual range [19]. In patients with a baseline Phe tolerance of ≤ 500 mg/day, Phe intake was increased weekly by 50 mg/day, in patients with a baseline Phe tolerance of >500 mg/day, Phe intake was increased weekly by 100 mg/day (Fig. 1). Increase of dietary Phe intake was performed in ve consecutive steps: 1. Low protein bread was replaced by "normal" bread. 2. Low protein pasta was replaced by "normal" pasta. 3. Milk and dairy products were included. 4. Meat and sausages were included. 5. Additionally, sh and eggs were included in the diet schedule. The intake of the amino acid formula was adapted weekly according to the actual individual Phe intake. In patients with a suf cient intake of natural protein by diet amino acid formula was stopped.

2.4. Installing BH4 treatment

BH4 was started in a dose of 20 mg/kg/day in all patients. In patients, who could stop Phe-restricted diet and amino acid supplementation, BH4 was reduced slowly, in steps of 100 mg/day weekly to two-weekly, until reaching a nal dose of 5–10 mg/kg/day (Fig. 1). In patients, who still received small amounts of amino acid formula, BH4 was slowly titrated by not adapting BH4 doses to the increasing weight. However, BH4 doses were only reduced if Phe levels were kept within the recommended range according to the patient's age and the patient's individual range [19]. Initially, 6RBH4 was applied (Schircks Laboratories, Switzerland); since 2009 BH4 is available with EMEA approval as the synthetic formulation sapropterin dihydrochloride (Kuvan®, Merck Serono, Germany). 2/18 patients also participated in the PKU-003 and PKU-004 study [4,5], 3/18 in the PKU-006 study [6], 4/18 patients have been reported in parts before [11].

None of the patients received additional permanent medication. Patients and their parents were asked for side effects every 3 months. In case of severe side effects, patients and their parents were advised to contact us immediately.

2.5. Laboratory analyses

During the initiation of BH4 treatment, plasma Phe was determined once to twice a week until reaching the individual nal Phe tolerance on BH4 treatment. After the phase of initiation, Phe was determined at least fortnightly to three-weekly, according to the patient's age [19]. Plasma Phe and Tyr were routinely determined by HPLC analyses (Agilent 1100 HPLC, Agilent Technologies, USA).

Venous blood sampling was performed in 4 h fasting state before start of BH4 treatment and every 6 months on BH4 treatment. Analyses included blood count, serum iron status, serum vitamin B12, plasma amino acid pro le, and plasma carnitine status. Additionally, methylmalonic acid was determined in urine.

PAH genotype had been determined in all patients after diagnosis, as previously described [20]. Mutations identi ed in the patients were analyzed for their potential BH4 responsiveness by comparing them with data published in http://www.biopku.org/biopku.

2.6. Predictive parameters

Long-term BH4 responders and long-term BH4 non-responders were compared according to their maximal Phe plasma concentration and their maximal Phe/tyrosine (Tyr) ratio before start of Phe-restricted diet and on Phe-restricted diet, their Phe tolerance at the age of 3 years [21], their results of neonatal BH4 loading test, and their genotype. These variables were used to compare the predictive value for long-term BH4 responsiveness.

2.7. Statistics

For statistical analyses IBM SPSS, Version 20.0, was used. Differences between patients groups were analyzed by the Mann–Whitney U Test. For graphic presentation of the data box plots were used.

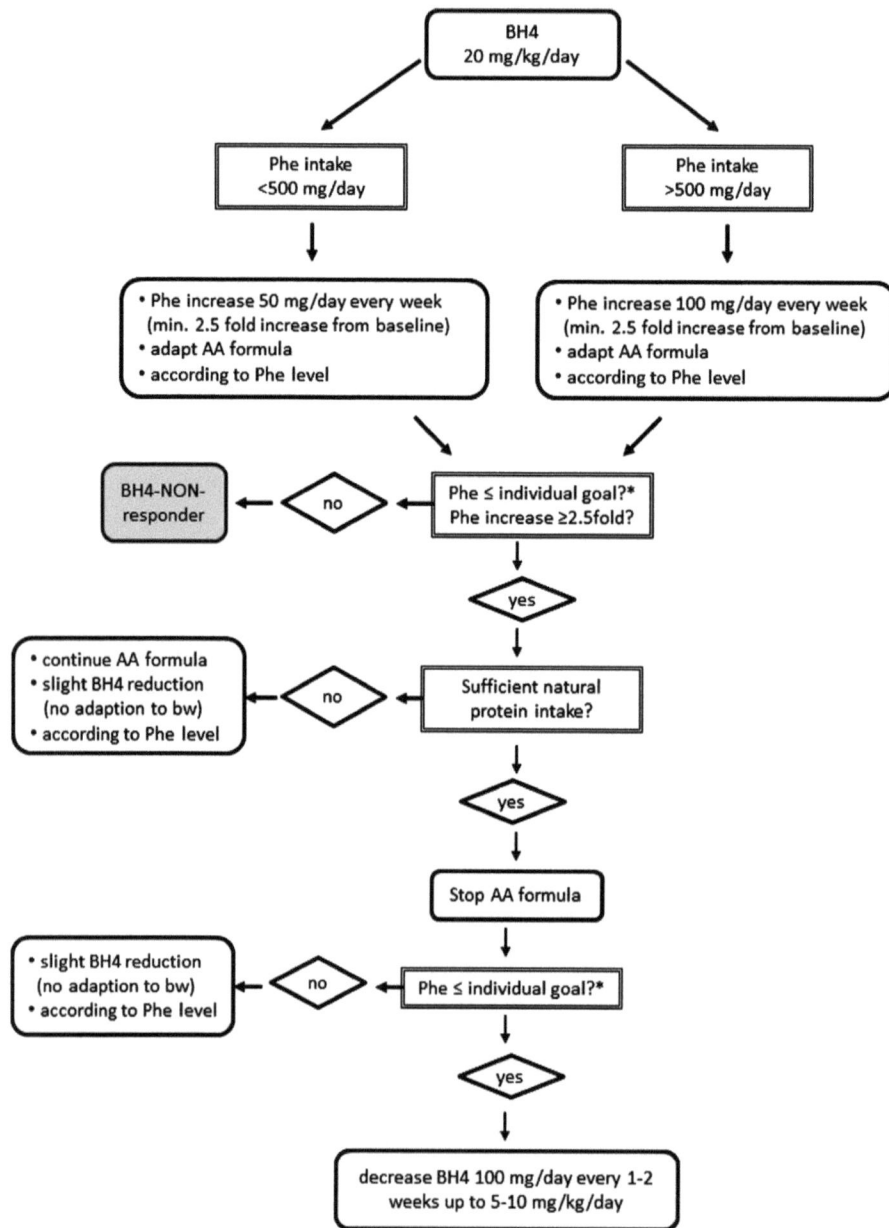

Table 1
Effects of BH4 treatment in long-term BH4 responders. Data on the individual final Phe tolerance and amino acid supplementation on BH4 long-term treatment, on the time needed to reach the individual final Phe tolerance, and on the actual BH4 dose.

ID	Final Phe tolerance (mg/day)	Increase in Phe tolerance	AA supplementation (g protein/kg/day)	Time needed to reach final Phe tolerance (weeks)	BH4 dose (mg/kg/day)
1	1100	5.8-fold	0.5	n.a.	18
2	2000	3.1-fold	0	6.4	14
3	2000	4.0-fold	0.4	35.9[a]	13
4	2000	3.3-fold	0	25.7	9
5	2400	5.5-fold	0	5.9	8
6	2000	3.6-fold	0	51.3[a]	15
7	880	2.5-fold	0.6	16.4	18
8	800	2.9-fold	0.8	n.a.	17
9	2000	3.1-fold	0	21.0	14
10	650	2.6-fold	0.9	n.a.	16
11	2600	2.7-fold	0.2	n.a.	17
12	2500	6.3-fold	0	8.3	12
13	1200	4.3-fold	0.6	35.9	18
14	1800	7.5-fold	0.6	n.a.	18
15	1600	2.7-fold	0	6.9	11
16	1600	2.7-fold	0	9.3	15
17	750	2.5-fold	0.8	15.0	19
18	800	2.7-fold	0.8	11.0	18

AA, amino acid formula.
n.a., not applicable: patients participated in the PKU-003, PKU-004, or PKU-006 study [4–6].
[a] Two patients had difficulties to sufficiently increase their Phe intake on long-term BH4 treatment. In both patients, time to reach their final Phe tolerance was delayed by the individual avoidance of protein-rich food.

3. Results

3.1. Long-term BH4 responsive patients

Out of 116 patients, only 24 patients were eligible for the start of long-term BH4 treatment. One patient refused treatment with BH4 due to optimal metabolic control on Phe-restricted diet. Of the remaining 23 patients, 12 were females and 11 males with a median age of 10.4 ± 4.3 years.

Out of these 23 patients, only 18 patients showed long-term response to BH4. In the remaining five patients, long-term BH4 treatment was stopped due to missing response, i.e. due to a failure of increasing Phe tolerance. Those 18 patients on long-term BH4 treatment were treated over a period of 48 ± 27 months (range: 8–105 months). In total, we collected data of cumulative 76 patient-years on long-term BH4 treatment.

3.2. Diet on long-term BH4 treatment

Clinical examination including weight and height revealed no abnormalities in any patient. In patients with long-term BH4 response, Phe tolerance was increased from 452 ± 201 mg/day (range: 190–960 mg/day) to 1593 ± 647 mg/day (range: 650–2600 mg/day), corresponding to a mean increase of 1141 ± 528 mg/day ($275 \pm 151\%$). In 8/18 patients, diet was completely liberalized; 10/18 patients still needed a Phe-free amino acid formula in a dose of 0.63 ± 0.23 g protein/kg/day. Final Phe tolerance was reached after 19.1 ± 14.2 weeks. However, there was a wide range within our study group: some patients reached their final Phe tolerance within a few weeks, whereas other patients needed several months to reach their final Phe tolerance (Table 1).

Increase of Phe intake as proposed by our protocol was well accepted by our patients and their parents. This protocol with a "slow" increase in Phe intake allowed the patients to get slowly acquainted with the change in diet with introduction of new food and new flavor. 2/18 patients on long-term BH4 treatment had difficulties to sufficiently increase their Phe intake, as they were well adapted to the Phe-restricted diet and refused protein-rich food. Well accepted protein-rich foods in all patients were normal bread, normal pasta, eggs, sausages and meat. In contrast, milk and dairy products were poorly accepted, and fish was completely refused by all patients.

Dietary protocols revealed no deficiencies in protein or calorie intake. However, on long-term BH4 treatment calcium intake were below daily recommendations [22] in 8/18 patients, vitamin B12 intake in 5/18 patients, and iron intake in 2/18 patients. Only patients on liberalized diet without additional amino acid intake revealed deficient intake in vitamins or micronutrients. All patients were extremely compliant to the prescribed Phe intake.

3.3. Long-term BH4 treatment

Mean BH4 dose on long-term treatment was 14.9 ± 3.3 mg/kg/day (range: 8.0–18.8 mg/kg/day). In patients on liberalized diet without additional amino acid intake BH4 dose was reduced to 12.2 ± 2.8 mg/kg/day (range: 8.0–15.4 mg/kg/day), in patients on amino acid supplementation median BH4 intake was 17.1 ± 1.6 mg/kg/day (range: 13.2–18.8 mg/kg/day). Absolute maximum daily BH4 dose was 1400 mg in one adolescent obese patient.

No severe side effects were reported on long-term BH4 treatment. Though, 7/18 patients reported minor side effects on long-term BH4 treatment: four patients were complaining about the taste of BH4, two patients about nausea after the intake of BH4 in the morning and one patient about recurrent abdominal pain. Quality of life was not examined by standardized questionnaires, but patients and parents were asked for subjective changes on BH4 treatment every 6 months. All patients reported of a positive effect of BH4 treatment by liberalizing dietary Phe restriction. In spite of side effects compliance to BH4 treatment was guaranteed by the positive effects of diet liberalization.

Fig. 1. Flow sheet for establishing BH4 treatment in patients with potential BH4 long-term responsiveness. Increase of Phe intake, adaption of amino acid formula and adaption of BH4 dose are indicated in the flow sheet. Patients with increasing Phe plasma concentrations above the individual goal and patients with insufficient increase of Phe intake were defined as BH4 non-responders. * Individual goal of plasma Phe concentrations were defined according to the age, the German recommendations and the individual patient's range. AA, amino acid formula; bw, body weight.

3.4. Laboratory parameters on long-term BH4 treatment

Life-long Phe plasma concentrations were available in all patients. Plasma Phe was analyzed regularly, according to the German recommendations for the treatment in PKU [19]. On BH4 treatment, Phe plasma levels did not change and stayed within individual ranges. Tyr plasma levels stayed within normal ranges as well.

Except an increase in Phe, plasma amino acid analyses revealed no further abnormalities. Plasma carnitine status, serum iron status, serum concentrations of vitamin B12, and urinary methylmalonic acid remained within normal values in all patients.

3.5. Parameters predicting long-term BH4 responsiveness

3.5.1. Phe plasma concentrations and Phe tolerance

Maximal Phe plasma concentration and maximal Phe/Tyr ratio before start of Phe-restricted dietary treatment and on Phe-restricted dietary treatment differed significantly between long-term BH4 responders and non-responders (Figs. 2A, B; Figs. 3A, B). In contrast, Phe tolerance, determined at the age of 3 years, did not differ significantly between both groups (25.6 ± 9.8 mg/kg/day in long-term BH4 responders; 17.9 ± 4.5 mg/kg/day in long-term BH4 non-responders). Most significant between both groups was the difference in maximal pretreatment plasma Phe concentrations.

3.5.2. BH4 loading test

Data of neonatal BH4 loading tests were available in 21/23 patients: in 7/21 patients only over a period of 8 h and in 14/21 patients over 24 h. Neonatal BH4 loading test was positive in 12/16 long-term BH4 responders (75%) and in 2/5 non-responders (40%). The 8 h BH4 loading was positive in 6/16 long-term BH4 responders (38%) and in 1/5 non-responders (20%); in contrast, the 24 h loading was positive in 11/12 long-term BH4 responders (92%) and in all non-responders (n = 2).

3.5.3. PAH genotype

PAH genotype analyses revealed one putative BH4 responsive mutation in 9/18 (50%) and two putative BH4 responsive mutations in 8/18 (44%) long-term BH4 responders. In one patient with long-term BH4 responsiveness only one mutation was identified. 4/5 long-term BH4 non-responders carried one putative BH4 responsive mutation (80%), none of them two putative BH4 responsive mutations. In one patient with long-term BH4 non-responsiveness a new missense mutation, p.V399A, was identified (Tables 2A and 2B).

3.5.4. Predictive values

Calculating all parameters for determining the potential of long-term BH4 responsiveness most predictive value was the combination of a pretreatment maximum plasma Phe concentration of b 1200 mol/L, a pretreatment maximum Phe/Tyr ratio of b 15, a maximum Phe/Tyr ratio of b 15 on dietary treatment, a Phe tolerance of > 20 mg/kg/day at the age of 3 years, a positive neonatal BH4 loading test, and a putative BH4 responsive genotype (p = 0.00024). Calculating only those parameters available shortly after diagnosing the patients in the neonatal period, i.e. the combination of a pretreatment maximum plasma Phe concentration of b 1200 mol/L, a pretreatment maximum Phe/Tyr ratio of b 15, a positive neonatal BH4 loading test, and a putative BH4 responsive PAH genotype was still significantly different between long-term BH4 responders and non-responders (p = 0.02). There was no significant difference between the occurrence of one or of two BH4 responsive alleles in predicting long-term BH4 responsiveness.

4. Discussion

Although BH4 treatment has been reported already more than 10 years ago [2], guidelines for installing BH4 treatment and for identifying long-term BH4 responders are not established yet.

Many studies focused on the effect of BH4 on blood Phe levels [4,5,14], but our data show that an increase in Phe tolerance might be an excellent outcome parameter for determining long-term BH4 responsiveness. Starting long-term BH4 treatment in patients with PKU requires strict dietary control. We could demonstrate an effective method by stepwise increasing Phe intake and exchanging low protein food with "normal food", associated with an excellent compliance of the patients and their parents. However, PKU patients develop special food habits, and some protein-rich food is rarely accepted by PKU patients who had been on a Phe-restricted diet before. In some patients on liberalized diet without additional intake of amino acid formula, vitamins and micronutrients must be supplemented [10].

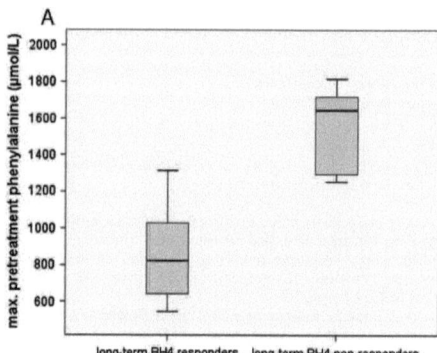

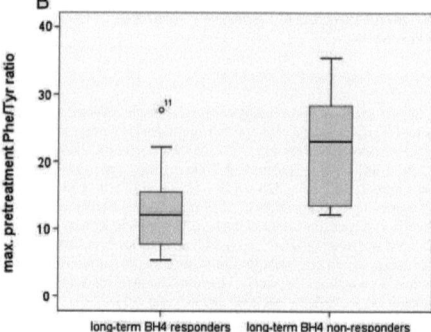

Fig. 2. A: Maximum pretreatment Phe plasma levels in BH4 long-term responders and non-responders. Maximum pretreatment Phe plasma levels were 849 ± 240 mol/L in BH4 long-term responders (n = 18) and 1546 ± 255 mol/L in BH4 long-term non-responders (n = 5). Maximum pretreatment Phe was significantly lower in BH4 long-term responders (p = 0.0003). B: Maximum pretreatment Phe/Tyr ratio in BH4 long-term responders and non-responders. Maximum pretreatment Phe/Tyr ratios were 12.4 ± 6.5 in BH4 long-term responders (n = 18) and 22.5 ± 9.9 in BH4 long-term non-responders (n = 5). Maximum pretreatment Phe/Tyr ratio was significantly lower in BH4 long-term responders (p = 0.048).

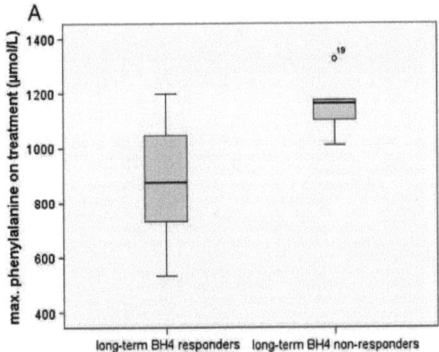

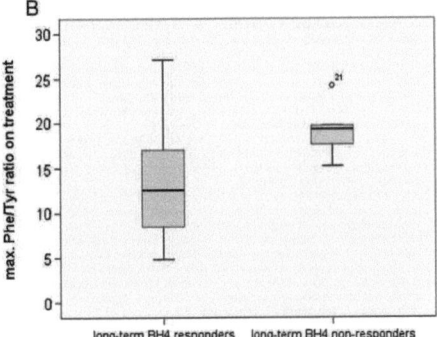

Fig. 3. A: Maximum Phe plasma levels in BH4 long-term responders and non-responders on Phe-restricted diet. Maximum Phe plasma levels on treatment were 876±187 μmol/L in BH4 long-term responders (n=18) and 1155±115 μmol/L in BH4 long-term non-responders (n=5). Maximum Phe on treatment was significantly lower in BH4 long-term responders (p=0.007). B: Maximum Phe/Tyr ratio in BH4 long-term responders and non-responders on Phe-restricted diet. Maximum Phe/Tyr ratios on treatment were 13.3±6.1 in BH4 long-term responders (n=18) and 19.2±3.3 in BH4 long-term non-responders (n=5). Maximum Phe/Tyr ratio on treatment was significantly lower in BH4 long-term responders (p=0.03).

Recently, it has been reported that many BH4 responsive *PAH* variants are in need for higher doses of BH4 [23]. This was confirmed by our data, revealing a need for BH4 doses of at least 15 mg/kg/day in the majority of the patients, particularly in patients still needing amino acid supplementation. Lower BH4 doses were only effective in a few patients with a mild PKU phenotype. No severe side effects of long-term BH4 treatment were reported in our patients, especially any thrombocytopenia, as recently reported [24]. Nevertheless, one third of the patients on long-term BH4 treatment complained of unpalatability and gastrointestinal side effects. In contrast to a previous study [9], all patients confirmed an increase in quality of life when starting BH4 treatment.

The identification of long-term BH4 responders still raises difficulties. Although we included only patients with a mild phenotype, a putative BH4 responsive *PAH* genotype and/or a positive neonatal BH4 loading, only 78% of these patients showed long-term BH4 responsiveness.

Biochemical parameters including maximum Phe levels and Phe/Tyr ratio were helpful in differentiating long-term BH4 responders

Table 2A
Genotype in long-term BH4 responders.

ID	Genotype	
	Allele 1	Allele 2
1	p.Y414C[a]	p.R408W
2	IVS11-8G>A	p.A403V[a]
3	p.R408W	p.R68S[b]
4	p.E390G[a]	p.E390G[a]
5	p.D129G[a]	p.R408W
6	p.Y414C[a]	p.A104D[b]
7	p.R408W	n.i.
8	p.P281L[b]	p.R261Q[b]
9	p.A403V[a]	p.R158Q[b]
10	p.R261Q[b]	p.R261Q[b]
11	p.R408W	p.I48S[a]
12	p.I306V[a]	p.I65T[b]
13	p.Y414C[a]	p.R252W
14	p.A395P[a]	p.Y414C[a]
15	p.I48S[a]	p.I48S[a]
16	p.R408W	p.K320N[a]
17	p.V190A[a]	p.S231F
18	IVS10-11G>A[b]	p.I65T[b]

n.i., not identified.
[a] BH4 responsive mutation.
[b] Variant BH4-responsive mutation.

and non-responders. However, Phe tolerance at age 3 years did not differ significantly between long-term BH4 responders and non-responders. This might be caused by potential inaccuracies in determining Phe tolerance by home-monitoring, and not by standardized in-patient conditions.

Various BH4 loading tests for identifying BH4 responders have been described; however, both, negative and positive false BH4 responders have been reported, e.g. due to late BH4 responsiveness, a low BH4 dose, a missing Phe challenge, a lack of compliance or catabolism [25,26]. Most interfering factors are more likely to disturb BH4 loading in older patients than in neonates. The neonatal BH4 loading test is currently routinely performed in neonates diagnosed with PKU only in Europe, except for the UK and Sweden, and in western Canada. Our data show that the neonatal BH4 loading test seems to be one good predictive parameter for determining long-term BH4 responsiveness. However, slow responders may be missed by the 24 h neonatal BH4 loading, and an extension to at least 48 h BH4 loading must be considered [27].

Currently, more than 600 *PAH* mutations are known, and more than 400 different mutation combinations have been reported in BH4 responsive PKU (18, http://www.biopku.org/biopku). Nevertheless, our data show that mutation analyses alone does not reliably predict long-term BH4 responsiveness. BH4 responsiveness seems to be consistent in certain genotypes, but inconsistent in other genotypes. Inconsistency with BH4 responsiveness in some genotypes has been explained by interallelic complementation [28]. Interallelic complementation may

Table 2B
Genotype in long-term BH4 non-responders.

ID	Genotype	
	Allele 1	Allele 2
19	p.I65T[b]	IVS4-5G>T
20	p.R408W	p.A309V[a]
21	p.R408W	p.I348V[b]
22	p.R408W	p.V399A[c]
23	p.R408W	p.R261Q[b]

[a] BH4 responsive mutation.
[b] Variant BH4-responsive mutation.
[c] Newly identified mutation.

occur in a compound heterozygote state, when the gene product is less or more active than the gene product of the homozygote mutations. As about 75% of the *PAH* genotypes are compound heterozygote, this may be of particular importance in patients with PKU [28]. Furthermore, it has been shown that variant *PAH* mutations may present with different BH4 responses according to their second mutation in trans: e.g. p.R261Q has been reported to be associated with BH4 responsiveness if occurring in homozygosity, whereas p.R261Q occurring in heterozygosity with a null mutation is not associated with BH4 responsiveness [23]. This may explain why one of our patients with homozygosity for p.R261Q showed long-term BH4 responsiveness, whereas one patient with compound heterozygosity for p.R261Q did not.

The newly identified missense mutation p.V399A is localized in a highly conserved region in the C-terminal region, i.e. in the catalytic domain (http://genome.ucsc.edu). Therefore, it is very likely that p.V399A is associated with a severe PKU phenotype und with unresponsiveness to BH4.

Our data show that no single parameter was specific enough to predict long-term BH4 responsiveness. We could indentify clinical, biochemical and genetic parameters which may predict long-term BH4 responsiveness. Those parameters which are already available soon after diagnosis of PKU in the neonatal period (pretreatment maximum Phe concentration, pretreatment Phe/Tyr ratio, neonatal BH4 loading test and *PAH* genotype) are still significant enough to predict long-term BH4 responsiveness. This may help in considering treatment options and in counseling soon after diagnosis.

Many factors influence BH4 responsiveness, including the actual metabolic control. Even if patients respond in the BH4 loading test, the long-term effect of BH4 treatment may be lacking. In contrast, long-term BH4 responders may show a negative result in the BH4 loading test, even in neonatal period. Furthermore, long-term BH4 treatment may increase PAH stability and the chaperone effect of BH4 [23]. Therefore, we recommend an extended BH4 treatment to reliably test individual BH4 responsiveness in well selected PKU patients with potential long-term BH4 responsiveness. As our data show, these patients may be selected by clear defined clinical, biochemical, and genetic parameters.

Considering the incomplete long-term BH4 response of a relevant part of PKU patients and the costs of a combined treatment with BH4 and Phe restricted diet, we recommend a strict indication of long-term BH4 treatment. Our data confirm that mainly patients with a milder phenotype may significantly benefit from long-term BH4 treatment. In patients with a more severe phenotype, Phe tolerance may only be increased in small amounts. It remains debatable if BH4 should be applied if Phe tolerance cannot be increased at least 2.5fold or even more. This is in accordance to previous data on the effect of long-term BH4 treatment [10]. Definitely, guidelines managing long-term BH4 treatment in PKU patients are needed.

5. Conclusion

Best predictive parameters for predicting long-term BH4 responsiveness seem to be the maximum pretreatment Phe plasma concentration and Phe/Tyr ratio, a positive neonatal BH4 loading test and at least one putative BH4 responsive *PAH* mutation. Mainly patients with a milder PKU phenotype may benefit from the long-term treatment with BH4. A clear defined protocol with stepwise increase of dietary Phe intake has been shown to be an effective strategy in long-term BH4 treatment.

Conflicts of interest

JBH, SR, and CG received contracts from Merck Serono, Germany. This study was supported by Merck Serono, Germany.

References

[1] C.R. Scriver, S. Kaufman, Phenylalanine hydroxylase deficiency, in: C.R. Scriver, A.L. Beaudet, W. Sly, D. Valle, B. Childs, B. Vogelstein (Eds.), The Metabolic and Molecular Basis of Inherited Disease, 8th ed., McGraw-Hill, New York, 2001, pp. 1667-1724.
[2] S. Kure, D.C. Hou, T. Ohura, H. Iwamoto, S. Suzuki, N. Sugiyama, O. Sakamoto, K. Fujii, Y. Matsubara, K. Narisawa, Tetrahydrobiopterin-responsive phenylalanine hydroxylase deficiency, J. Pediatr. 135 (1999) 375-378.
[3] A.C. Muntau, W. Röschinger, M. Habich, H. Demmelmair, B. Hoffmann, C.P. Sommerhoff, A.A. Roscher, Tetrahydrobiopterin as an alternative treatment for mild phenylketonuria, N. Engl. J. Med. 347 (2002) 2122-2132.
[4] H.L. Levy, A. Milanowski, A. Chakrapani, M. Cleary, P. Lee, F.K. Trefz, C.B. Whitley, F. Feillet, A.S. Feigenbaum, J.D. Bebchuk, H. Christ-Schmidt, A. Dorenbaum, Sapropterin Research Group, Efficacy of sapropterin dihydrochloride (tetrahydrobiopterin, 6R-BH4) for reduction of phenylalanine concentration in patients with phenylketonuria: a phase III randomised placebo-controlled study, Lancet 11 (370) (2007) 504-510.
[5] P. Lee, E.P. Treacy, E. Crombez, M. Wasserstein, L. Waber, J. Wolff, U. Wendel, A. Dorenbaum, J. Bebchuk, H. Christ-Schmidt, M. Seashore, M. Giovannini, B.K. Burton, A.A. Morris, Sapropterin Research Group, Safety and efficacy of 22 weeks of treatment with sapropterin dihydrochloride in patients with phenylketonuria, Am. J. Med. Genet. 146A (2008) 2851-2859.
[6] F.K. Trefz, B.K. Burton, N. Longo, M.M. Casanova, D.J. Gruskin, A. Dorenbaum, E.D. Kakkis, E.A. Crombez, D.K. Grange, P. Harmatz, M.H. Lipson, A. Milanowski, L.M. Randolph, J. Vockley, C.B. Whitley, J.A. Wolff, J. Bebchuk, H. Christ-Schmidt, J.B. Hennermann, Sapropterin Study Group, Efficacy of sapropterin dihydrochloride in increasing phenylalanine tolerance in children with phenylketonuria: a phase III, randomized, double-blind, placebo-controlled study, J. Pediatr. 154 (2009) 700-707.
[7] F.K. Trefz, D. Scheible, G. Frauendienst-Egger, Long-term follow-up of patients with phenylketonuria receiving tetrahydrobiopterin treatment, J. Inherit. Metab. Dis. (2010, Mar 9. [Epub ahead of print]) (PMID: 20217238).
[8] A. Burlina, N. Blau, Effect of BH(4) supplementation on phenylalanine tolerance, J. Inherit. Metab. Dis. 32 (2009) 40-45.
[9] B. Ziesch, J. Weigel, A. Thiele, U. Mütze, C. Rohde, U. Ceglarek, J. Thiery, W. Kiess, S. Beblo, Tetrahydrobiopterin (BH4) in PKU: effect on dietary treatment, metabolic control, and quality of life, J. Inherit. Metab. Dis. (2012 Mar 6. [Epub ahead of print]) (PMID: 22391997).
[10] R.H. Singh, M.E. Quirk, T.D. Douglas, M.C. Brauchla, BH(4) therapy impacts the nutrition status and intake in children with phenylketonuria: 2-year follow-up, J. Inherit. Metab. Dis. 33 (2010) 689-695.
[11] J.B. Hennermann, C. Bührer, N. Blau, B. Vetter, E. Mönch, Long-term treatment with tetrahydrobiopterin increases phenylalanine tolerance in children with severe phenotype of phenylketonuria, Mol. Genet. Metab. 86 (2005) S86-S90.
[12] C. Bernegger, N. Blau, High frequency of tetrahydrobiopterin-responsiveness among hyperphenylalaninemias: a study of 1,919 patients observed from 1988 to 2002, Mol. Genet. Metab. 77 (2002) 304-313.
[13] M.R. Zur Ühh, J. Zschocke, M. Lindner, F. Feillet, C. Chery, A. Burlina, R.C. Stevens, B. Thöny, N. Blau, Molecular genetics of tetrahydrobiopterin-responsive phenylalanine hydroxylase deficiency, Hum. Mutat. 29 (2008) 167-175.
[14] B.K. Burton, D.K. Grange, A. Milanowski, G. Vockley, F. Feillet, E.A. Crombez, V. Abadie, C.O. Harding, S. Cederbaum, D. Dobbelaere, A. Smith, A. Dorenbaum, The response of patients with phenylketonuria and elevated serum phenylalanine to treatment with oral sapropterin dihydrochloride (6R-tetrahydrobiopterin): a phase II, multicentre, open-label, screening study, J. Inherit. Metab. Dis. 30 (2007) 700-707.
[15] A. Cunningham, H. Bausell, M. Brown, M. Chapman, K. DeFouw, S. Ernst, J. McClure, H. McCune, D. O'Steen, A. Pender, J. Skrabal, A. Wessel, E. Jurecki, R. Shediac, S. Prasad, J. Gillis, S. Cederbaum, Recommendations for the use of sapropterin in phenylketonuria, Mol. Genet. Metab. 106 (2012) 269-276.
[16] P. Guldberg, F. Rey, J. Zschocke, V. Romano, B. Francois, L. Michiels, K. Ullrich, G.F. Hoffmann, P. Burgard, H. Schmidt, C. Meli, E. Riva, I. Dianzani, A. Ponzone, J. Rey, F. Güttler, A European multicenter study of phenylalanine hydroxylase deficiency: classification of 105 mutations and a general system for genotype-based prediction of metabolic phenotype, Am. J. Hum. Genet. 63 (1998) 71-79.
[17] F. Güttler, K.F. Guldberg, Mutations in the phenylalanine hydroxylase gene: genetic determinants for the phenotypic variability of hyperphenylalaninemia, Acta Paediatr. 407 (Suppl.) (1994) 46-56.
[18] N. Blau, J.B. Hennermann, U. Langenbeck, U. Lichter-Konecki, Diagnosis, classification, and genetics of phenylketonuria and tetrahydrobiopterin (BH4) deficiencies, Mol. Genet. Metab. 104 (Suppl.) (2011) S2-S9.
[19] P. Burgard, H.J. Bremer, P. Bührdel, P.C. Clemens, E. Mönch, H. Przyrembel, F.K. Trefz, K. Ullrich, Rationale for the German recommendations for phenylalanine level control in phenylketonuria 1997, Eur. J. Pediatr. 158 (1999) 46-54.
[20] J.B. Hennermann, C. Wolf, E. Windt, P. Bührdel, J. Seidel, E. Mönch, A.E. Kulozik, Phenylketonuria and hyperphenylalaninemia in Eastern Germany: a characteristic molecular profile and 15 novel mutations, Hum. Mutat. 15 (2000) 254-260.
[21] F.J. van Spronsen, M. van Rijn, B. Dorgelo, M. Hoeksma, A.M. Bosch, M.F. Mulder, J.B.C. de Klerk, T. de Koning, M. Estela Rubio-Gozalbo, M. de Vries, P.H. Verkerk, Phenylalanine tolerance can already reliably be assessed at the age of 2 years in patients with PKU, J. Inherit. Metab. Dis. 32 (2009) 27-31.
[22] D-A-CH Empfehlung: Deutsche Gesellschaft für Ernährung, Österreichische Gesellschaft für Ernährung, Schweizerische Gesellschaft für Ernährungsforschung, Schweizerische Vereinigung für Ernährung, 2000 (Referenzwerte für die Nährstoffzufuhr: Umschau/Braus).
[23] M. Staudigl, S.W. Gersting, M.K. Danecka, D.D. Messing, M. Woidy, D. Pinkas, K.F. Kemter, N. Blau, A.C. Muntau, The interplay between genotype, metabolic state

and cofactor treatment governs phenylalanine hydroxylase function and drug response, Hum. Mol. Genet. 20 (2011) 2628–2641.
[24] B.K. Burton, M. Nowacka, J.B. Hennermann, M. Lipson, D.K. Grange, A. Chakrapani, F. Trefz, A. Dorenbaum, M. Imperiale, S.S. Kim, P.M. Fernhoff, Safety of extended treatment with sapropterin dihydrochloride in patients with phenylketonuria: results of a phase 3b study, Mol. Genet. Metab. 103 (2011) 315–322.
[25] N. Blau, A. Bélanger-Quintana, M. Demirkol, F. Feillet, M. Giovannini, A. MacDonald, F.K. Trefz, F.J. van Spronsen, Optimizing the use of sapropterin (BH(4)) in the management of phenylketonuria, Mol. Genet. Metab. 96 (2009) 158–163.
[26] J.B. Nielsen, K.E. Nielsen, F. Güttler, Tetrahydrobiopterin responsiveness after extended loading test of 12 Danish PKU patients with the Y414C mutation, J. Inherit. Metab. Dis. 33 (2010) 9–16.
[27] B. Fiege, L. Bonafé, D. Ballhausen, M. Baumgartner, B. Thöny, D. Meili, L. Fiori, M. Giovannini, N. Blau, Extended tetrahydrobiopterin loading test in the diagnosis of cofactor-responsive phenylketonuria: a pilot study, Mol. Genet. Metab. 86 (Suppl. 1) (2005) S91–S95.
[28] J. Leandro, P. Leandro, T. Flatmark, Heterotetrameric forms of human phenylalanine hydroxylase: co-expression of wild-type and mutant forms in a bicistronic system, Biochim. Biophys. Acta 1812 (2011) 602–612.

2.7. PUBLIKATION 7: Blau N, **Hennermann JB**, Langenbeck U, Lichter-Konecki U. Diagnosis, Classification, and Genetics of Phenylketonuria and Tetrahydrobiopterin (BH4) Deficiencies. 2011. Mol Genet Metab 104:S2-S9. DOI 10.1016/j.ymgme. 2011.08.017

Reprinted from: Molecular Genetics and Metabolism 2011, Volume 86 Suppl, page S2-9, with permission from Elsevier Inc., 2011, provided by Copyright Clearance Center

Abschließend fasst dieser Artikel das derzeitige Wissen, die neuen Entwicklungen sowie häufige Schwierigkeiten bei Diagnosestellung, Klassifizierung und genetischen Analysen aller Störungen im Phe-Stoffwechsel, d. h. sowohl des PAH-Mangels wie auch der Störungen in der BH4-Synthese und -Regeneration, zusammen. Alle Patienten, die im Neugeborenenscreening mittels Tandem-Massenspektrometrie mit einer Phe-Erhöhung auffallen, müssen auf eine Störung der BH4-Synthese und -Regeneration untersucht werden. Aus einer einzigen Trockenblutkarte können sowohl die Analyse der Aminosäuren Phe und Tyr als auch die Analyse der Pterine (Neopterin und Biopterin) sowie die Aktivität der Dihydropteridin-Reduktase durchgeführt werden. Nach der Diagnosestellung empfiehlt sich baldmöglichst eine Klassifizierung der Patienten in den jeweiligen PKU-Phänotyp. Der PKU-Phänotyp wird durch die Phe-Blutwerte und durch die tägliche individuelle Phe-Toleranz bestimmt, aber auch durch ein potentielles Ansprechen auf BH4. Nach den aktuellen Empfehlungen sollte der BH4-Belastungstest mit der Gabe von synthetischem BH4, Sapropterin, in einer Dosierung von 20 mg/kg/Tag durchgeführt werden. Nach einem initialen Screening Test über einen Zeitraum von 24-48 Stunden sollte der BH4-Test über mehrere Wochen fortgeführt werden. Anhand des Genotyps, d. h. anhand der Kombination der Mutationen beider PAH-Allele, kann die Schwere der PKU, d. h. der biochemische Phänotyp, aber auch ein potentielles Ansprechen auf BH4 leichter bestimmt werden. Zudem kann mit einer Phe-Belastung und der hierbei erzielten Phe-Umsetzungsrate der PKU-Phänotyp sicher klassifiziert werden.

Die Einteilung in die verschiedenen PKU-Phänotypen und die Klassifizierung des *PAH*-Genotyps ist essentiell für mögliche Therapie-Entscheidungen, insbesondere der Therapie mit BH4, sowie für eine adäquate Beratung der betroffenen Familien.

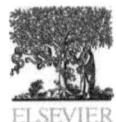
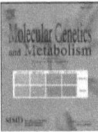

Molecular Genetics and Metabolism

journal homepage: www.elsevier.com/locate/ymgme

Minireview

Diagnosis, classification, and genetics of phenylketonuria and tetrahydrobiopterin (BH4) deficiencies

Nenad Blau [a,b,c,*], Julia B. Hennermann [d], Ulrich Langenbeck [e], Uta Lichter-Konecki [f]

[a] University Children's Hospital, Zürich, Switzerland
[b] Zürich Center for Integrative Human Physiology (ZIHP), Zürich, Switzerland
[c] Research Center for Children (RCC), Zürich, Switzerland
[d] Department of Pediatrics, Charité Universitätsmedizin Berlin, Germany
[e] Institute of Human Genetics, University Hospital, Frankfurt/Main, Germany
[f] Center for Neuroscience and Behavioral Medicine, Division of Genetics & Metabolism, Children's National Medical Center, Department of Pediatrics, George Washington University, Medical Center, Washington, DC, USA

article info

Article history:
Received 8 July 2011
Received in revised form 17 August 2011
Accepted 17 August 2011
Available online 26 August 2011

Keywords:
Phenylketonuria
PKU
BH4
Tetrahydrobiopterin

abstract

This article summarizes the present knowledge, recent developments, and common pitfalls in the diagnosis, classification, and genetics of hyperphenylalaninemia, including tetrahydrobiopterin (BH4) deficiency. It is a product of the recent workshop organized by the European Phenylketonuria Group in March 2011 in Lisbon, Portugal. Results of the workshop demonstrate that following newborn screening for phenylketonuria (PKU), using tandem mass-spectrometry, every newborn with even slightly elevated blood phenylalanine (Phe) levels needs to be screened for BH4 deficiency. Dried blood spots are the best sample for the simultaneous measurement of amino acids (phenylalanine and tyrosine), pterins (neopterin and biopterin), and dihydropteridine reductase activity from a single specimen. Following diagnosis, the patient's phenotype and individually tailored treatment should be established as soon as possible. Not only blood Phe levels, but also daily tolerance for dietary Phe and potential responsiveness to BH4 are part of the investigations. Efficiency testing with synthetic BH4 (sapropterin dihydrochloride) over several weeks should follow the initial 24–48-hour screening test with 20 mg/kg/day BH4. The specific genotype, i.e. the combination of both *PAH* alleles of the patient, helps or facilitates to determine both the biochemical phenotype (severity of PKU) and the responsiveness to BH4. The rate of Phe metabolic disposal after Phe challenge may be an additional useful tool in the interpretation of phenotype–genotype correlation.

© 2011 Elsevier Inc. All rights reserved.

Contents

1. Diagnosis S3
   1.1. Newborn screening S3
   1.2. Differential diagnosis S3
   1.3. BH4 loading test S3
   1.4. Cerebrospinal fluid investigation S4
2. Classification S4
   2.1. Phenylalanine loading test S4
   2.2. Phenotypes S5
   2.3. Blood phenylalanine S5
   2.4. Phenylalanine tolerance S5
   2.5. Clinical course S5
   2.6. Software and phenylalanine home monitoring device S5

Abbreviations: BH4, tetrahydrobiopterin; CNS, central nervous system; DHPR, dihydropteridine reductase; DBS, dried blood spot; HPA, hyperphenylalaninemia; KOUT, 1st order rate of metabolic disposal; MHP, mild HPA; PAH, phenylalanine hydroxylase; PBW, percent body weight; PKU, phenylketonuria; PROT, net protein synthesis; TMS, tandem mass-spectrometry.
* Corresponding author at: University Children's Hospital, Steinwiesstrasse 75 8032 Zürich, Switzerland.
E-mail addresses: nenad.blau@kispi.uzh.ch (N. Blau), julia.hennermann@charite.de (J.B. Hennermann), ulrich.langenbeck@gmx.net (U. Langenbeck), ulichter@childrensnational.org (U. Lichter-Konecki).

1096-7192/$ – see front matter © 2011 Elsevier Inc. All rights reserved.
doi:10.1016/j.ymgme.2011.08.017

3. Genetics S6
   3.1. PAH mutations and PKU genotypes (incl. databases) S6
   3.2. Phenotype–genotype correlation S6
   3.3. BH4-responsive mutations and genotypes S7
Acknowledgments. S7
References S8

1. Diagnosis

1.1. Newborn screening

Phenylketonuria (PKU) is identified through national newborn screening programs [1]. The first efficient test for hyperphenylalaninemia (HPA) was a bacterial inhibition assay developed by Robert Guthrie [2]. The test was based on *Bacillus subtilis*, which requires phenylalanine (Phe) for growth. The Guthrie test was very useful for mass screening as the dried blood spot (DBS) can be obtained in the hospital or a doctor's office using a standardized filter paper ("Guthrie card") and mailed to reference laboratories in an envelope. Tandem mass-spectrometry (TMS) was developed as a fast method for achieving reliable and quantitative determination of concentrations of amino acids in small volumes of blood or plasma [3]. This method provides a lower rate of false positive results, by measuring levels of both Phe and Tyr and providing the Phe/Tyr ratio, and thus requires fewer resources to follow up such cases. In addition, other inborn errors of metabolism can be identified simultaneously.

All infants should be screened for PKU within the first days of life, in order to allow timely dietary intervention to protect children with PKU from neurological damage. Where screening is carried out in maternity wards, the blood sample is usually obtained between days 2 and 5; in general, however, screening is carried out mostly between the ages of 2 and 7 days [4]. In the U.S., samples are typically obtained at 24–48 h. A commonly used Phe cut-off level for diagnosis of PKU is 120–130 μmol/L (with a Phe/Tyr ratio >2), with TMS employed [5]. Concern has been expressed that screening too early, associated with a shift towards earlier discharge from maternity wards, can provide a false negative result, as there will have been insufficient opportunity for Phe from the diet to build up to diagnostic (and toxic) levels. It is currently accepted that the sensitivity of screening in a healthy neonate is adequate before 24 h of life, especially where the screening test involves measurement of Phe/Tyr ratios to increase sensitivity relative to Phe measurement alone [3,6]. However, as the pretreatment level is often used as a diagnostic parameter for the classification of the PKU phenotype new cut-offs have to be determined for classic and mild PKU and mild HPA when measuring the Phe level so early.

Some infants, particularly those born prematurely, may demonstrate immaturity of enzyme systems involved in amino acid metabolism, resulting in a transient elevation of blood Phe to a level sufficient to test positive in a PKU screening test. The results of early PKU screening should also be interpreted with caution in sick neonates or in neonates under parenteral nutrition or blood transfusion, and a second screening test should be sent if it is unclear whether the child had sufficient protein intake when the first test was collected.

1.2. Differential diagnosis

About 2% of all Phe level elevations detected by the newborn screening are due to disorders in BH4 metabolism, highlighting the importance of always considering the differential diagnosis for every even slightly elevated blood Phe level [7]. Frequency of BH4 deficiency is higher in some countries where the rate of consanguineous marriages tends to maintain the presence of genetic disorders within families, e.g. Turkey or Saudi Arabia [8]. BH4 deficiencies are more severe than PKU with regard to their response to therapy and treatment is substantially different. Low-Phe diet is not effective and early substitution with dopamine and serotonin precursors, as well as with the synthetic BH4 (sapropterin dihydrochloride) is crucial for a good outcome. Analysis of DBS or urine for neopterin and biopterin and measurement of dihydropteridine reductase (DHPR) activity in the DBS is essential for the exact diagnosis and should be performed as early as possible. A BH4 loading test and measurement of neurotransmitter metabolites, pterins, and folates in cerebrospinal fluid add further important information about the severity of the disease [9].

In patients with BH4 deficiency, the pattern of pterins is identical in blood, urine, and CSF. The use of DBS on filter paper (Guthrie card) is, however, more practical and allows measurement of pterins, DHPR activity, and amino acids from a single specimen [10]. It is important to know that patients with classic PKU excrete more pterins in urine compared with healthy controls and the amount of excreted metabolites is directly proportional to blood Phe levels. Diseases that cause activation of the immune system (elevated neopterin), and anticancer therapy or rheumatic disease therapy with methotrexate (inhibition of DHPR), may interfere with the analytic procedures. Some patients with DHPR deficiency show a normal blood or urinary neopterin and biopterin profile. Therefore, DHPR activity measurement is essential in all patients with HPA, regardless of pterin measurements. Fig. 1 shows the algorithm for the diagnostic work-up of elevated blood Phe levels. Table 1 summarizes the most important biochemical parameters used in the differential diagnosis of HPA.

1.3. BH4 loading test

The BH4 loading test was initially used to discriminate between patients with elevated phenylalanine levels due to PAH deficiency and patients with elevated Phe levels due to BH4 deficiency (enzyme defects in the biosynthesis or regeneration of the cofactor BH4) [11,12]. Thus, the loading test is an additional useful tool for the early detection of BH4 deficiencies and it was used in Europe for almost 30 years. In addition, this test detects PKU patients responsive to BH4 administration.

Detection of BH4-responsive PKU patients is important because some PKU patients benefit from oral administration of BH4 (sapropterin dihydrochloride) in that their blood Phe level decreases or even normalizes under pharmacological therapy with BH4 [13]. The phenomenon of BH4-sensitive PKU was initially described in Japanese patients, and confirmed in retrospective and prospective studies with large cohorts of patients [14–16]. Modalities of the BH4 challenge vary in the literature from a 24-hour test with a single administration of BH4 (10–20 mg/kg) to several weeks of administration with daily or weekly monitoring of blood Phe levels [17,18].

There is general agreement that a reduction on blood Phe of at least 30% in response to BH4 loading indicates a clinically significant effect, although in some centers a lower cut-off value may be defined for individual patients, or no specific cut-off value may be used [19]. The frequency of BH4-responsiveness is highest in patients with mild (non-PKU) HPA, or mild PKU resulting from *PAH* mutations that allow for residual enzyme activity [15,20]. Conversely, the response rate among patients with classic PKU (little or no residual

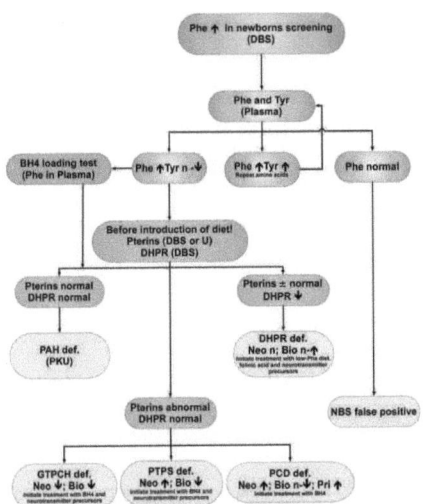

Fig. 1. Diagnostic flow-chart for the laboratory diagnosis of PKU and BH4 deficiencies. Modified according to Opladen et al. [10]. Dried blood spots (DBS) or random urine (U) can be used for the differential diagnosis depending on the profile of neopterin (Neo), biopterin (Bio), and primapterin (Pri) and dihydropteridine reductase (DHPR) activity in DBS, diagnosis of following BH4 deficiencies can be established: GTP cyclohydrolase I (GTPCH) deficiency (low or no detectable neopterin and biopterin), 6-pyruvoyl-tetrahydropterin synthase (PTPS) deficiency (high neopterin and low or no detectable biopterin), dihydropteridine reductase (DHPR) deficiency (normal neopterin and normal or elevated biopterin and no DHPR activity), and pterins-4a-carbinolamine dehydratase (PCD) deficiency (elevated neopterin, low-normal biopterin, and elevated primapterin). n: normal.

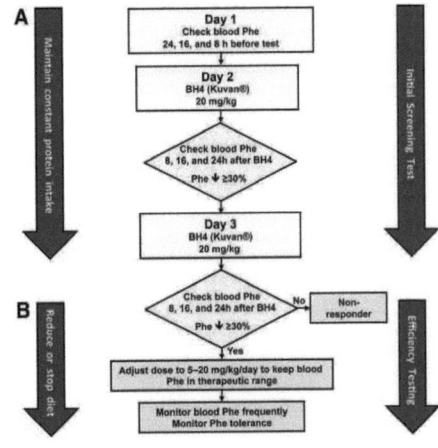

Fig. 2. Proposed algorithms for the BH4 (sapropterin dihydrochloride) challenge, screening, and initiating treatment in BH4-responsive PKU patients. A) Initial screening test with blood Phe monitoring on the first day and BH4 (sapropterin dihydrochloride) administration (20 mg/kg) on two following days; B) Efficiency testing in BH4-responsive patients over several weeks with BH4 doses adjusted individually according to Phe tolerance and therapeutic blood Phe levels.

PAH activity) is very low. A number of *PAH* mutations associated with BH4 responsiveness have been identified and genotyping is a useful additional tool for predicting responsiveness [21,22] (see below). Fig. 2 summarizes the proposed procedure for the BH4 loading test in Europe. In newborns the test should be performed before introducing the low-Phe diet and at elevated blood Phe levels (>400 μmol/L). In infant or adult PKU patients on a Phe-restricted diet, the diet needs to be modified by increasing the protein intake (egg or milk powder before and during the test). Table 2 summarizes factors that may potentially influence the outcome of the test.

An international online survey [23] with 92 participants from 30 different countries documented that in 62% of the metabolic centers the BH4 loading test is an integral part of the diagnostic work-up for PKU. The main reason for not using the BH4 test is either relatively high costs or no availability of BH4 in some countries (78%). Most centers use the BH4 test in all age groups (79%) and only in about 11% of the metabolic centers pregnant PKU women are tested. A dosage of 20 mg/kg is used in 92% of the centers and duration of the test is quite variable: 24 h (33%), 48 h (24%), 72 h (16%), and about 26% run the test over 1–4 weeks, most of them from the U.S. with test duration over at least 4 weeks. About half of the survey participants defined BH4-responsiveness as both increase in tolerance for dietary Phe (by a factor of two) and reduction in blood Phe levels (by at least 30%), while the rest use only blood Phe reduction as criterion.

1.4. Cerebrospinal fluid investigation

BH4 deficiency influences the synthesis of catecholamines, serotonin [24] and nitric oxide [25] in the central nervous system (CNS), and measurement of their metabolites in cerebrospinal fluid (CSF) is important for the diagnosis of different forms (severe v. mild) of BH4 deficiencies. Not only the absolute levels of 5-hydroxyindoleacetic acid and homovanillic acid in CSF, but also differences in the ratios of neurotransmitter levels provide important diagnostic information relating to the severity and outcome of BH4 deficiency [26].

2. Classification

2.1. Phenylalanine loading test

Phenylalanine loading tests were applied since 1956 for the detection of heterozygotes in PKU families [27], until, in the late 1980s, this

Table 1
Biochemical parameters in dried blood spots (DBS) used in the differential diagnosis of PKU and BH4 deficiencies.

Deficiency	Neopterin	Biopterin	Primapterin	DHPR activity	Phe
PKU	n-↑	n-↑	n	n	↑
GTPCH	↓	↓	n	n	↑[a]
PTPS	↑	↓	n	n	↑
PCD	↑	↓-n	↑	n	↑
DHPR	n	n-↑[a]	n	↓	↑

[a] Can be normal in the early neonatal period.

Table 2
Factors potentially affecting the BH4 loading test.

- BH4 dosage (higher sensitivity with 20 mg/kg v. 10 mg/kg)
- Duration of the test (24–48 h for initial screening v. 4–8 weeks for efficiency)
- Food intake (better GI absorption of BH4 with high calories food)
- Age (outcome may be different in newborns v. adolescents v. adults)
- Diet (better response to BH4 when out of diet and on higher blood Phe levels)
- GI absorption (may be individually different; monitor blood BH4 levels)
- Genotype

approach was replaced by molecular analysis of *PAH* gene haplotypes and mutations [28]. Phenylalanine loading tests gained further interest when Guthrie card mass screening uncovered not only the expected cases of classic PKU but also variants of PKU [29]. Because these variants were initially thought not to require dietary treatment, a reliable discrimination of these phenotypes was needed. For practical and ethical reasons, *in vivo* ^{3}H or ^{14}C isotope studies [30] or invasive testing such as enzyme assays from liver biopsies [31] were not appropriate. Therefore, Blaskovics [32] developed in the mid-1960s the standardized three day natural protein loading test with evaporated milk that was applied at 6 months of age in the U.S. [33] and German [34] PKU Collaborative Studies for classification of PKU and for genotype-phenotype analysis. With this test three principal types of Phe blood level response, types 1, 2 and 3, were delineated in both studies. Type 1 is characterized by a 72 h Phe beyond 1200 μmol/L and corresponds to classic PKU. Type 2 is defined by a spontaneous decline of Phe levels, despite continuation of loading, from above 1200 μmol/L after day 2 to a 72 h Phe levels of 1200–600 μmol/L. In both studies, about 10% of the patients belong to this type. In type 3 the plasma Phe fluctuates around 600 μmol/L and the 72 h Phe levels are <600 μmol/L. Clinically, it corresponds to mild HPA. On a free diet, these patients (22% in the U.S., and 13% in the German study) do not need a low-Phe treatment for normal mental outcome [35].

Major successes of the Blaskovics loading test were (i) the discovery of the type 2 response as an indicator of mutant enzyme activation by Phe [36], (ii) the delineation of the type 3 response as the base for the decision to discontinue dietetic treatment, and (iii) its use as a measure of *in vivo* phenotype for genotype–phenotype analysis. In contrast to its proven scientific value, the test has only limited value for the dietetic treatment of patients with classic and mild PKU because the Phe 72 value will not predict the current and future individual dietary requirements (see below) and the patients may manifest during the test signs of intoxication such as nausea, vomiting, irritability, insomnia and EEG changes. The test is no longer necessary [37] and has been replaced in practice by predictive molecular and enzymatic classifications [22,38]. A recent online survey accordingly revealed that only 4% of centers still use it for estimating the phenotype of their patients [23].

2.2. Phenotypes

Depending on the enzyme defect, the genotype and the severity of the disease, different forms of PKU with different clinical phenotypes have been described. Thus, different classifications for PKU phenotypes have been established. PKU may be classified as classic PKU and as variant PKU which includes all milder forms of PKU, (i.e. moderate PKU and mild PKU), as mild HPA or non-PKU HPA, and, additionally, as BH4-responsive PKU [29,39,40]. Definition of PKU phenotypes may be essential in establishing treatment options, e.g. new therapeutic strategies, in counseling and in prediction of the outcome, and in pregnancy. Pretreatment blood Phe levels, the individual Phe tolerance, and the clinical course of the disease may help to discriminate the different phenotypes of PKU, but are not precise parameters and the cut-offs for pretreatment levels collected during the first 24–48 h, as they relate to the different types of PKU, have to be newly defined.

2.3. Blood phenylalanine

In 1980, for the first time, blood Phe levels were used to discriminate between three different phenotypes of PKU [29]. Still, this classification of the various types of PAH deficiency is used for phenotyping PKU: Classic PKU is defined by presenting with Phe pretreatment levels >1200 μmol/L, variant PKU with Phe pretreatment levels of 600–1200 μmol/L and mild HPA with Phe pretreatment levels <600 μmol/L. More precisely, PAH deficiency may be classified into four different phenotypes: classic PKU presenting with Phe pretreatment levels >1200 μmol/L, moderate PKU with Phe pretreatment levels of 900–1200 μmol/L, mild PKU with Phe pretreatment levels of 600–900 μmol/L, and mild HPA with Phe pretreatment level <600 μmol/L [38,39].

Although pretreatment Phe levels are indispensable for phenotyping PKU, they are dependent on some variables, e. g. on the timing of blood Phe measurement, on the neonatal catabolism, and on the diet received at the time of blood sampling. Due to improvement in newborn screening with an early blood sampling at day three of life, patients with PKU are diagnosed much earlier, thus resulting in significantly lower pretreatment Phe levels. If pretreatment Phe levels will be used for determining PKU phenotypes in the future, this classification needs to be adjusted. In day-to-day-practice, pretreatment blood Phe levels have been shown to be used for phenotyping patients with PKU in about 80% of the treatment centers [23].

2.4. Phenylalanine tolerance

Daily Phe tolerance has been established as a stable parameter for phenotyping the various types of PAH deficiency [29]. Phe tolerance is usually determined at the age of 5 years and indicates the amount of daily Phe intake that a patient can tolerate without an increase of the blood Phe level above the upper target range. Three different phenotypes may be classified by using Phe tolerance: classic PKU with a Phe tolerance <20 mg/kg/day, variant PKU with a Phe tolerance of 20–50 mg/kg/day, and mild HPA with a Phe tolerance >50 mg/kg/day [29]. More detailed is the classification into four different phenotypes, who defines classic PKU with a Phe tolerance <20 mg/kg/day (250–300 mg/day), moderate PKU with a Phe tolerance of 20–25 mg/kg/day (350–400 mg/day), mild PKU with a Phe tolerance of 25–50 mg/kg/day (400–600 mg/day), and mild HPA with patients off diet [38,39].

Recently it has been shown that Phe tolerance may be predictable already at the age of 2 years, and that Phe tolerance at age 2, 3, and 5 years correlates with that at age 10 years [41]. In contrast, reassessment of Phe tolerance may be necessary in adults [42]. Although Phe tolerance is a good indicator for the PKU phenotype, its determination may be unreliable if not determined under standardized conditions. In day-to-day-practice, prescribed Phe intake often is much lower than the effective Phe intake at home. We therefore recommend determining Phe tolerance under standardized in-patient conditions with precise dietary protocols. In clinical follow-up, Phe tolerance is used for phenotyping patients with PKU in 70% of metabolic centers queried [21].

2.5. Clinical course

Furthermore, various types of PAH deficiency may be distinguished by the clinical course of the disease. This includes data on the outcome (e. g. education, IQ), the maximum blood Phe concentrations (e. g. during febrile infection, dietary non-compliance), the fluctuation of blood Phe levels, and the Phe/Tyr ratios [43,44]. Though, in day-to-day-practice, clinical course of the disease is only used in 31% of metabolic centers to distinguish different PKU forms [23].

In day-to-day practice, classification of PKU is essential for choosing the optimal treatment. This may suggest a simplified classification scheme based on treatment requirements: a) patients who do need strict dietary treatment (PKU), b) patients who do not need any treatment (non-PKU HPA), c) patients who may be treated with BH4 (BH4-responsive PKU).

2.6. Software and phenylalanine home monitoring device

The Blaskovics loading tests at 6 months with their resulting 72 h Phe values [32] yield indicators of metabolic phenotypes which belong to a bimodal distribution with nadir at about 1,200 and 1,600 μmol/L, respectively [33,34], thus establishing a classification into classic and variant PKU. A more detailed separation of the metabolic phenotypes was established by Güttler and Guldberg [45] through estimating Phe tolerance at 5 years of age (see also above). Neither of these systems can, at any age, predict the individual Phe tolerance. This is made possible, however, by mathematical analysis of the data with a kinetic model using per cent body water (PBW), net protein synthesis (PROT), and 1st order rate of metabolic disposal (KOUT) of Phe as variable parameters [46]. Both PBW and PROT are age-dependent parameters, whereas KOUT is expected not to change with age. With age-specific PBW and PROT data from the literature [47], an age-independent KOUT would enable the reliable prediction of evolution of Phe tolerance at all ages. Even in adults, from their Blaskovics test data, provided the patients, or their data, can be 'retrieved' again [48].

By kinetic analysis of the protein loading data of the German PKU Study it has been possible to explain the type 2 response as a consequence of mutant PAH activation by high Phe levels [36]. Also some mild cases, originally classified as type 1, were found to be activated by Phe levels to some extent. The distribution of the KOUT estimates, including the maximal KOUT estimates of the cases with activation, is depicted in Fig. 3. This distribution is apparently multimodal and the peaks appear to represent classic (a), moderate (b), and mild PKU (c), and mild HPA (d), respectively. These findings can be compared to the classification of Güttler and Guldberg [45] by treating the dietary tolerance at the target Phe level as the equilibrium state of Phe metabolism. In the kinetic model [46] this corresponds to:

$$\text{Target Phe} = ((\text{intake}-\text{PROT})\text{mg=day})=\text{PBW} * \text{KOUT=day} \quad (1)$$

With Eq. (1) and taking PBW = 0.65 and PROT = 2.7 mg Phe per kg body weight and day, the classification of Güttler and Guldberg translates into KOUT values of 0.62 and 1.08 per day for moderate and mild PKU, respectively. The data at KOUT = 1.7 (d) corresponds within this system to an equilibrium Phe level of 110 μmol/L at an intake of 120 mg Phe per kg body weight and day (here taken as 'normal diet').

These calculations implicate that the constant of metabolic disposal of Phe is about identical between 6 months and 5 years of age and may therefore be considered as a patient-specific parameter. This is relevant for the day-to-day management of PKU children, because it has been shown (in an observational study) that increased Phe values, in a considerable part of cases, are the consequence of hidden catabolism (as indicated in the model by diminished PROT values) and not of non-compliance [49].

Application of this kinetic model in a user-friendly format (e.g. a so-called App) would support self-control with home-monitoring devices [50] and could be trained e.g. in PKU summer camps. Such a device is presently in development and according to a recent survey [23], 85% would consider home monitoring of Phe useful for both children and pregnant women.

3. Genetics

3.1. PAH mutations and PKU genotypes (incl. databases)

As already stated, knowing whether a patient has residual PAH enzyme activity can be relevant for the therapeutic approach, the likely Phe tolerance, and the expected response to BH4. Delineation of the mutations of the PAH gene was initiated immediately after the cloning of the gene in 1983 [28]. Initially the most prevalent mutations in the Western European population were identified and characterized with regard to the in vitro residual enzyme activity associated with the respective mutation [51,52]. Subsequently a 'Phenylalanine Hydroxylase Locus Knowledgebase' PAHdb was created and curated at McGill University [53] (http://www.pahdb.mcgill.ca/) that cataloged knowledge about PAH alleles and mutations and their characteristics as reported by clinicians and laboratories from around the world. This database now lists a total of 564 PAH mutations discovered world wide as well as the knowledge available about the respective mutation including the residual enzyme activities of ~200 mutations. Of the 564 mutations 60.5% are missense mutations, 13.5% deletions, 11% splice site mutations, (5.7% silent mutations), 5% nonsense mutations, and 1.8% insertions. It was evident early on that the majority of the PAH mutations were missense mutations not preventing transcription or translation and that the majority of the patients are compound heterozygotes, meaning they carry a different mutation in each of their alleles. PAH deficiency thus most often results from complex interactions of mutant alleles or rapid intracellular destruction of mutant enzyme subunits making genotype/phenotype correlations based on the knowledge about individual mutations challenging.

3.2. Phenotype–genotype correlation

The first publication with extensive data on genotype/phenotype correlation in PKU was able to establish that the genotype of the patient correlates with the biochemical phenotype [54]. PKU patients had been tested for 8 mutations of the PAH gene for which the in vitro residual enzyme activity had been determined. This mutation analysis had allowed for complete genotype determination (identifying both mutations) in 104 patients with PAH deficiency. Stringent classification criteria for the biochemical phenotype were applied to determine genotype/phenotype correlation in these 104 patients. There was a highly significant correlation between the genotype of the patients and the biochemical phenotype (r = 0.74–0.84, p<0.001 depending on the parameter) although the genotype was expressed as the predicted residual enzyme activity of the patient and was calculated as the mean of the combined in vitro residual enzyme activities of both mutant alleles of the patient, which was quite a simplification compared to the real in vivo situation. The goal of the research had been to determine whether genotype analysis after exclusion of BH4 cofactor deficiency could replace more involved clinical testing such as response to a standardized oral protein load at 6 months of age and Phe tolerance assessment in an inpatient setting over the course of 1–2 weeks at 5 years of age. These clinical tests had proven to be the most reliable clinical classification criteria in large

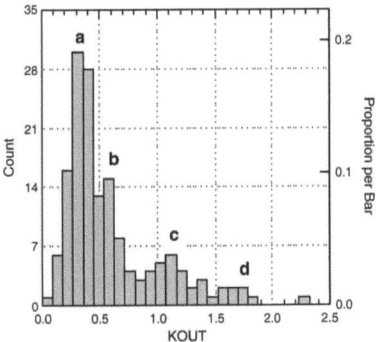

Fig. 3. Distribution of KOUT [per day], the 1st order rate constant of metabolic disposal of Phe, in the German PKU Study [36], N = 157. The data suggest the peaks a, b, c, and d as representing classic, moderate and mild PKU, and mild HPA, respectively. The apparently multimodal distribution implies a frequency in the German population of 15% and 8% for mild PKU and mild HPA. Normal KOUT values, determined by i.v. loads, range from 10.6 to 24.9 per day, corresponding to a half-life of 0.7 to 1.6 h.

clinical studies [54] but were cumbersome and in the case of the loading test exposed the patient to high Phe concentrations.

In 1998 Guldberg et al. [38] reported the identification of the complete genotype in 686 patients from 7 European centers. Based on the Phe tolerance (or in the case of mild HPA the pretreatment level) of 297 functionally hemizygous patients (patients carrying a null allele and the uncharacterized mutant allele), an arbitrary phenotype category was assigned to each of 105 mutations for which the residual enzyme activity was not known. Using these arbitrary categories phenotype predictions for 650 of the patients were made. In 79% of the patients the predicted phenotype matched the observed phenotype and the authors concluded that differences in the phenotype classification across centers might have accounted for the genotype–phenotype inconsistencies that were observed. Overall, despite the potential shortcomings, this work also led to the conclusion that the genotype is the main determinant of the biochemical phenotype in most patients with PAH deficiency.

Many more studies were published reporting genotype/phenotype correlations in different populations and inconsistencies, i.e. genotypes that were associated with several different phenotypes. It was also pointed out in numerous publications (first by S. Kaufman [55]) and investigated in vitro [56] that the combination of the two mutant alleles is important for the residual PAH enzyme activity and that the individual mutations of a patient should not be viewed by themselves. It is clear that the residual activity of an enzyme that is a homotetramer that consists of a combination of different mutant subunits may not simply be the mean of the activity that each subunit produces by itself in vitro because there may be negative intra-allelic complementation between different mutant enzyme subunits [55]. However, a correlation between genotype and biochemical phenotype prevailed in the majority of the patients reported. Limitations regarding genotype-based prediction of the phenotype, however, are that the in vitro residual enzyme activity is not known for all mutations, that negative intra-allelic complementation may occur, and some exceptions described below may occur.

3.3. BH4-responsive mutations and genotypes

As mentioned above a 'Phenylalanine Hydroxylase Locus Knowledgebase' PAHdb exists at McGill University [53] (http://www.pahdb.mcgill.ca/) that has catalogued knowledge about PAH alleles and mutations including the associated phenotype. It lists the phenotype associated with about 600 allele combinations; however this data is 'self-reported' by clinicians and laboratories using variable criteria for the determination of the phenotype. Another database, the BIOPKU database (www.biopku.org) was created at the University of Zürich. It has catalogued the complete genotypes (complete mutation combinations) of 730 PKU patients, their phenotypes (based on the highest blood Phe levels before starting treatment) and their response to BH4. These 730 patients represent a total of 430 different mutation combinations.

Some of the mutation combinations of the 730 patients listed are not always associated with the same phenotype. Mutations for which inconsistencies regarding genotype/phenotype correlation are reported in this database as well as in the literature are the R261Q mutation in the homozygous state or in combination with the R158Q mutation, the L48S mutation in the homozygous state or in combination with the R158Q mutation, and the Y414C mutation in combination with the R408W mutation. However, although different phenotypes are associated with these mutation combinations their BH4 responsiveness is always the same except in a smaller percentage of L48S homozygotes (19%) that may not respond while 81% respond. A similar phenomenon was observed in 40% of Turkish patients that were homozygous for the E390G mutation and did not respond to BH4 [22] while other homozygous patients and all patients compound heterozygous for this very mild mutation listed in the BIOPKU database did respond to BH4. The observations regarding variability for two mild mutations in the homozygous state indicate that certain mutant homotetramers may not allow for stable active enzyme even if the mutations themselves appeared to be mild in vitro. Patients homozygous for these particular mutations may occasionally not respond to BH4 or not within 48 h. Finally, for the c.1066-11G>A mutation in the homozygous state different phenotypes and the whole spectrum of BH4 responsiveness (negative, positive, and slow) is cataloged. Given that this is a mutation in an intron that creates a cryptic splice acceptor site it is conceivable that the cryptic splice site does not always come into play and functional enzyme is being translated under certain circumstances creating this variability.

General truths about genotype/phenotype correlations in PKU that have emerged from the data cataloged in the data bases, especially in the BIOPKU data base are:

1. Mutation combinations that allow for <15% in vitro enzyme activity cause classic PKU and do not respond to BH4. Mutation combinations that allow for >20% residual activity responds to BH4. Responders have moderate to mild phenotypes.
2. Splice site mutations may cause classic or mild PKU depending on 'read through' (i.e. normal splicing may sometimes occur despite the mutation), and the fact that they have different phenotype associations is listed in the available data bases.
3. Specific mild mutation/classic mutation combinations with identical predicted residual enzyme activity may have different phenotype associations (due to negative intra-allelic complementation) but the phenotype associations of different mutation combinations can be found in the available data bases making prediction unnecessary.
4. The BH4 responsiveness of many mutation combinations (complete genotypes) has been well established multiple times. Patients that have those genotypes may not need to undergo BH4 responsiveness testing.

After assessment of the genotype (both mutations) of a patient one can now in many cases simply look up the associated phenotype and BH4 responsiveness that is cataloged for this mutation combination in the databases rather than trying to predict it using a simplifying formula and the in vitro residual enzyme activity of the mutant alleles as was done in the past and had its limitations (see above). DNA diagnostic laboratories should include the information cataloged in the data bases for a specific mutation combination in their reports about PAH mutations to clinicians to allow physicians to make the best informed decisions based on available information.

In an anonymous survey among 65 US metabolic centers 72% of the centers reported that they classify PKU patients into classic PKU, mild PKU, and mild HPA; 40% were ordering mutation testing on all of their patients 53% on some of their patients; 53% of the centers order genotype analysis, when they order it, to understand the phenotype of the patient; 72% order to provide the family with genetic information (multiple answers could be chosen); of those who do not order mutation analysis 40% said they had too little information about the meaning of the mutations (what phenotype to expect), 54% said they do not need mutation analysis to understand the phenotype of their patients, and 36% said the health insurance of their patients does not cover the testing; 20% of the centers said they order mutation analysis on each PKU patient that wants to try BH4 supplementation to see whether the patient should have residual enzyme activity (which would make it more likely that patient responds to BH4).

Acknowledgments

Authors would like to thank Serono Scientific International Foundation (SSIF) for supporting organization of the workshop on "Diagnosis, classification and genetics of PKU". This work was supported in part by the Swiss National Science Foundation grant no. 31003A-119982 (to NB). UL is grateful to the German Collaborative Study on

PKU for providing the study data whose analysis resulted in Ref. [36] and Fig. 3 of the present communication.

References

[1] J.L. Dhondt, Laboratory diagnosis of phenylketonuria, in: N. Blau (Ed.), PKU and BH4: Advances in Phenylketonuria and Tetrahydrobiopterin, SPS Verlagsgesellschaft, Heilbronn, 2006, pp. 161–179.
[2] R. Guthrie, A. Susi, A simple phenylalanine method for detecting phenylketonuria in large populations of newborn infants, Pediatrics 32 (1963) 338–343.
[3] D.H. Chace, J.E. Sherwin, S.L. Hillman, F. Lorey, G.C. Cunningham, Use of phenylalanine-to-tyrosine ratio determined by tandem mass spectrometry to improve newborn screening for phenylketonuria of early discharge specimens collected in the first 24 hours, Clin. Chem. 44 (1998) 2405–2409.
[4] M. Zaffanello, G. Zamboni, C. Maffeis, L. Tato, Neonatal birth parameters of positive newborns at PKU screening as predictors of false-positive and positive results at recall-testing, J. Med. Screen 10 (2003) 181–183.
[5] Phenylketonuria (PKU): screening and management, NIH Consens. Statement 17 (2000) 1–33.
[6] J.W. Eastman, J.E. Sherwin, R. Wong, C.L. Liao, R.J. Currier, F. Lorey, G. Cunningham, Use of the phenylalanine:tyrosine ratio to test newborns for phenylketonuria in a large public health screening programme, J. Med. Screen 7 (2000) 131–135.
[7] N. Blau, B. Thöny, R.G.H. Cotton, K. Hyland, Disorders of tetrahydrobiopterin and related biogenic amines, in: C.R. Scriver, A.L. Beaudet, W.S. Sly, D. Valle, B. Childs, B. Vogelstein (Eds.), The Metabolic and Molecular Bases of Inherited Disease, McGraw-Hill, New York, 2001, pp. 1725–1776.
[8] N. Blau, F.J. Van Spronsen, H.L. Levy, Phenylketonuria, Lancet 376 (2010) 1417–1427.
[9] N. Longo, Disorders of biopterin metabolism, J. Inherit. Metab. Dis. 32 (2009) 333–342.
[10] T. Opladen, B. Abu Seda, A. Rassi, B. Thöny, G.F. Hoffmann, N. Blau, Diagnosis of tetrahydrobiopterin deficiency using filter paper blood spots: further development of the method and 5 years experience, J. Inherit. Metab. Dis. 34 (2011) 819–826.
[11] H.C. Curtius, A. Niederwieser, M. Viscontini, A. Otten, J. Schaub, S. Scheibenreiter, H. Schmidt, Atypical phenylketonuria due to tetrahydrobiopterin deficiency. Diagnosis and treatment with tetrahydrobiopterin, dihydrobiopterin and sepiapterin, Clin. Chim. Acta 93 (1979) 251–262.
[12] A. Ponzone, O. Guardamagna, I. Dianzani, R. Ponzone, G.B. Ferrero, M. Spada, R.G.H. Cotton, Catalytic activity of tetrahydrobiopterin in dihydropteridine reductase deficiency and indications for treatment, Pediatr. Res. 33 (1993) 125–128.
[13] A.C. Muntau, W. Röschinger, M. Habich, H. Demmelmair, B. Hoffmann, C.P. Sommerhoff, A.A. Roscher, Tetrahydrobiopterin as an alternative treatment for mild phenylketonuria, N. Engl. J. Med. 347 (2002) 2122–2132.
[14] C. Bernegger, N. Blau, High frequency of tetrahydrobiopterin-responsiveness among hyperphenylalaninemias: a study of 1919 patients observed from 1988 to 2002, Mol. Genet. Metab. 77 (2002) 304–313.
[15] B. Fiege, N. Blau, Assessment of tetrahydrobiopterin (BH4)-responsiveness in phenylketonuria, J. Pediatr. 150 (2007) 627–630.
[16] H. Levy, A. Milanowski, A. Chakrapani, M. Cleary, P. Lee, F.K. Trefz, C.B. Whitley, F. Feillet, A.S. Feigenbaum, J.D. Bebchuk, H. Christ-Schmidt, A. Dorenbaum, Efficacy of sapropterin dihydrochloride (tetrahydrobiopterin, 6R-BH4) for reduction of phenylalanine concentration in patients with phenylketonuria: a phase III randomized placebo-controlled study, Lancet 370 (2007) 504–510.
[17] N. Blau, Sapropterin dihydrochloride for phenylketonuria and tetrahydrobiopterin deficiency, Expert. Rev. Endocrinol. Metab. 5 (2010) 483–494.
[18] H. Levy, B. Burton, S. Cederbaum, C. Scriver, Recommendations for evaluation of responsiveness to tetrahydrobiopterin (BH(4)) in phenylketonuria and its use in treatment, Mol. Genet. Metab. 92 (2007) 287–291.
[19] N. Blau, Defining tetrahydrobiopterin (BH4)-responsiveness in PKU, J. Inherit. Metab. Dis. 31 (2008) 2–3.
[20] B.K. Burton, D.K. Grange, A. Milanowski, G. Vockley, F. Feillet, E.A. Crombez, V. Abadie, C.O. Harding, S. Cederbaum, D. Dobbelaere, A. Smith, A. Dorenbaum, The response of patients with phenylketonuria and elevated serum phenylalanine to treatment with oral sapropterin dihydrochloride (6R-tetrahydrobiopterin): a phase II, multicentre, open-label, screening study, J. Inherit. Metab. Dis. 30 (2007) 700–707.
[21] M.R. Zurflüh, J. Zschocke, M. Lindner, F. Feillet, C. Chery, A. Burlina, R. Stevens, B. Thöny, N. Blau, Molecular genetics of tetrahydrobiopterin responsive phenylalanine hydroxylase deficiency, Hum. Mutat. 29 (2008) 167–175.
[22] S.T. Dobrowolski, C. Heintz, T. Miller, C.R. Ellingson, C.C. Ellingson, I. Özer, G. Gökcay, T. Baykal, B. Thöny, M. Demirkol, N. Blau, Molecular genetics and impact of residual in vitro phenylalanine hydroxylase activity on tetrahydrobiopterin-responsiveness in Turkish PKU population, Mol. Genet. Metab. 10 (2011) 116–121.
[23] N. Blau, U. Langenbeck, J.B. Hennermann, U. Lichter Konecki, Diagnosis and management of PKU: an international survey J Inherit Metab Dis (abstract), 34 (Suppl 3) (2011) S97.
[24] K. Hyland, R.A.H. Surtees, S.J.R. Heales, A. Bowron, D.W. Howells, I. Smith, Cerebrospinal fluid concentrations of pterins and metabolites of serotonin and dopamine in a pediatric reference population, Pediatr. Res. 34 (1993) 10–14.
[25] G. Zorzi, B. Thöny, N. Blau, Reduced nitric oxide metabolites in CSF of patients with tetrahydrobiopterin deficiency, J. Neurochem. 80 (2002) 362–364.
[26] L. Jäggi, M.R. Zurflüh, A. Schuler, A. Ponzone, F. Porta, L. Fiori, M. Giovannini, R. Santer, G.F. Hoffmann, H. Ibel, U. Wendel, D. Ballhausen, M.R. Baumgartner, N. Blau, Outcome and long-term follow-up of 36 patients with tetrahydrobiopterin deficiency, Mol. Genet. Metab. 93 (2008) 295–305.
[27] K.W. Driscoll, D.Y. Hsia, W.E. Knox, W Troll, Detection by phenylalanine tolerance tests of heterozygous carriers of phenylketonuria, Nature 178 (1956) 1239–1240.
[28] S.L. Woo, A.S. Lidsky, F. Güttler, T. Chandra, K.J. Robson, Cloned human phenylalanine hydroxylase gene allows prenatal diagnosis and carrier detection of classical phenylketonuria, Nature 306 (1983) 151–155.
[29] F. Güttler, Hyperphenylalaninemia: diagnosis and classification of the various types of phenylalanine hydroxylase deficiency in childhood, Acta Paediatr. Scand. Suppl. 280 (1980) 1–80.
[30] W.D. Lehmann, R. Fischer, H.C. Heinrich, P. Clemens, R. Grüttner, Metabolic conversion of L-[U-14 C]phenylalanine to respiratory 14CO2 in healthy subjects, phenylketonuria heterozygotes and classic phenylketonurics, Clin. Chim. Acta 157 (1986) 253–266.
[31] M.C. Hsieh, H.K. Berry, M.K. Bofinger, P.J. Phillips, M.B. Guilfoile, M.M. Hunt, Comparative diagnostic value of phenylalanine challenge and phenylalanine hydroxylase activity in phenylketonuria, Clin. Genet. 23 (1983) 415–421.
[32] M.E. Blaskovics, Phenylketonuria: loading studies revisited, in: N. Blau (Ed.), PKU and BH4: Advances in Phenylketonuria and Tetrahydrobiopterin, SPS Verlagsgesellschaft, Heilbronn, 2006, pp. 104–119.
[33] M.E. O'Flynn, N.A. Holtzman, M. Blaskovics, C. Azen, M.L. Williamson, The diagnosis of phenylketonuria: a report from the Collaborative Study of Children Treated for Phenylketonuria, Am. J. Dis. Child. 134 (1980) 769–774.
[34] P. Lutz, H. Schmidt, U. Batzler, Study design and description of patients, Eur. J. Pediatr. 149 (Suppl 1) (1990) S5–S12.
[35] J. Weglage, M. Pietsch, R. Feldmann, H.G. Koch, J. Zschocke, G. Hoffmann, A. Muntau-Heger, J. Denecke, P. Guldberg, F. Güttler, H. Möller, U. Wendel, K. Ullrich, E. Harms, Normal clinical outcome in untreated subjects with mild hyperphenylalaninemia, Pediatr. Res. 49 (2001) 532–536.
[36] U. Langenbeck, P. Burgard, U. Wendel, M. Lindner, J. Zschocke, Metabolic phenotypes of phenylketonuria. Kinetic and molecular evaluation of the Blaskovics protein loading test, J. Inherit. Metab. Dis. 32 (2009) 506–513.
[37] J. Donlon, H. Levy, C.R. Scriver, Hyperphenylalaninemia: phenylalanine hydroxylase deficiency, in: D. Valle, A.L. Beaudet, B. Vogelstein, K.W. Kinzler, S.E. Antonarakis, A. Ballabio (Eds.), The Online Metabolic & Molecular Bases of Inherited Disease, McGraw-Hill, Montreal, 2008, Ch. 77.
[38] P. Guldberg, F. Rey, J. Zschocke, V. Romano, B. Francois, L. Michiels, K. Ullrich, G.F. Hoffmann, P. Burgard, H. Schmidt, C. Meli, E. Riva, I. Dianzani, A. Ponzone, J. Rey, F. Güttler, A European multicenter study of phenylalanine hydroxylase deficiency: classification of 105 mutations and a general system for genotype-based prediction of metabolic phenotype, Am. J. Hum. Genet. 63 (1998) 71–79.
[39] P. Guldberg, F. Güttler, Mutations in the phenylalanine hydroxylase gene: methods for their characterization, Acta Paediatr. Suppl. 407 (1994) 27–33.
[40] S. Kure, D.C. Hou, T. Ohura, H. Iwamoto, S. Suzuki, N. Sugiyama, O. Sakamoto, K. Fujii, Y. Matsubara, K. Narisawa, Tetrahydrobiopterin-responsive phenylalanine hydroxylase deficiency, J. Pediatr. 135 (1999) 375–378.
[41] F.J. van Spronsen, M. van Rijn, B. Dorgelo, M. Hoeksma, A.M. Bosch, M.F. Mulder, J.B. de Klerk, T. de Koning, M.E. Rubio-Gozalbo, M. de Vries, P.H. Verkerk, Phenylalanine tolerance can already reliably be assessed at the age of 2 years in patients with PKU, J. Inherit. Metab. Dis. 32 (2009) 27–31.
[42] E.L. MacLeod, S.T. Gleason, S.C. van Calcar, D.M. Ney, Reassessment of phenylalanine tolerance in adults with phenylketonuria is needed as body mass changes, Mol. Genet. Metab. 98 (2009) 331–337.
[43] V. Anastasoaie, L. Kurzius, P. Forbes, S. Waisbren, Stability of blood phenylalanine levels and IQ in children with phenylketonuria, Mol. Genet. Metab. 95 (2008) 17–20.
[44] J. Humphrey, J. Nation, I. Francis, A. Boneh, Effect of tetrahydrobiopterin on Phe/Tyr ratios and variation in Phe levels in tetrahydrobiopterin responsive PKU patients, Mol. Genet. Metab. (2011), doi:10.1016/j.ymgme.2011.1005.1011.
[45] F. Güttler, P. Guldberg, The influence of mutations on enzyme activity and phenylalanine tolerance in phenylalanine hydroxylase deficiency, Eur. J. Pediatr. 155 (1996) S 6–S 10.
[46] U. Langenbeck, J. Zschocke, U. Wendel, V. Hönig, Modelling the phenylalanine blood level response during treatment of phenylketonuria, J. Inherit. Metab. Dis. 24 (2001) 805–814.
[47] S.J. Fomon, P. Haschke, E.E. Ziegler, S.E. Nelson, Body composition of reference children from birth to age 10 years, Am. J. Clin. Nutr. 35 (1982) 1169–1175.
[48] B.K. Burton, L. Leviton, Reaching out to the lost generation of adults with early-treated phenylketonuria (PKU), Mol. Genet. Metab. 101 (2010) 146–148.
[49] U. Langenbeck, M. Ammar, J. Zschocke, E. Solem, I.M. Knerr, J. Herwig, H. Boehles, Recognizing catabolic states during dietary treatment of phenylketonuria. An application of metabolic modelling J Inherit Metab Dis 34 (Suppl 3) (2011) S102.
[50] U. Wendel, U. Langenbeck, Towards self-monitoring and self-treatment in phenylketonuria—a way to better diet compliance, Eur. J. Pediatr. 155 (Suppl 1) (1996) S105–S107.
[51] D.S. Konecki, U. Lichter Konecki, The phenylketonuria locus: current knowledge about alleles and mutations of the phenylalanine hydroxylase gene in various populations, Hum. Genet. 87 (1991) 377–388.

[52] R.C. Eisensmith, Y. Okano, M. Dasovich, T. Wang, F. Güttler, H. Lou, P. Guldberg, U. Lichter-Konecki, D.S. Konecki, E. Svensson, et al., Multiple origins for phenylketonuria in Europe, Am. J. Hum. Genet. 51 (1992) 1355–1365.

[53] L. Hoang, S. Byck, L. Prevost, C.R. Scriver, PAH mutation analysis consortium database — a database for disease-producing and other allelic variation at the human PAH locus, Nucleic Acids Res. 24 (1996) 127–131.

[54] Y. Okano, R.C. Eisensmith, F. Güttler, U. Lichter-Konecki, D.S. Konecki, F.K. Trefz, M. Dasovich, T. Wang, K. Henriksen, H. Lou, et al., Molecular basis of phenotypic heterogeneity in phenylketonuria, N. Engl. J. Med. 324 (1991) 1232–1238.

[55] S. Kaufman, Phenylketonuria: Biochemical Mechanisms, in: B.W. Agranoff, M.H. Aprison (Eds.), Advances in Neurochemistry, Plenum Press, New York, 1976, pp. 1–132.

[56] P.J. Waters, How PAH gene mutations cause hyper-phenylalaninemia and why mechanism matters: insights from in vitro expression, Hum. Mutat. 21 (2003) 357–369.

3. Diskussion

3.1. Phenylalanin-bilanzierte diätetische Therapie

Seit Einführung des Neugeborenenscreenings auf PKU in Deutschland in den späten 1960er bzw. frühen 1970er Jahren werden Patienten mit einer PKU frühzeitig diagnostiziert und rechtzeitig behandelt. Das Outcome von PKU-Patienten ist jedoch abhängig von der individuellen Stoffwechseleinstellung: Ein Phe-Anstieg um 100 µmol/L in dem kritischen Alter der ersten 12 Lebensjahre bedingt einen Abfall des IQs um 1,3-3,1 Punkte, wie eine kürzlich durchgeführte Metaanalyse ergab (Waisbren et al. 2007).

Obwohl die Phe-bilanzierte Diät bereits in den 1950er Jahren erstmals beschrieben wurde, hat sich in der Behandlung der PKU und in der Zusammensetzung der diätetischen Therapie erst in den letzten Jahren einiges geändert. Wegen Complianceproblemen (MacDonald et al. 2010, Walter et al. 2002), Einschränkungen der Lebensqualität (Cotugno et al. 2011) und möglicher Langzeitfolgen durch die Phe-bilanzierte Diät begann die Suche nach neuen Optionen in der Behandlung der PKU.

3.1.1. Langzeitprobleme unter Phenylalanin-bilanzierter Diät

Mikronährstoff-Defizite, insbesondere ein Vitamin B12-Mangel, sind eines der möglichen Langzeitprobleme bei Patienten mit PKU. Dies betrifft jedoch vorwiegend Patienten mit ausgeprägter Incompliance, Patienten, die ihre diätetische Therapie ohne eine adäquate Proteinversorgung beenden, oder Patienten mit HPA und streng veganer Ernährung (MacDonald et al. 2011). Weitere bekannte Langzeitprobleme bei adoleszenten und adulten Patienten mit PKU sind Osteopenie bzw. Osteoporose (Hoeks et al. 2009, Schwahn et al. 1998) sowie neurologische Defizite, wie Tremor, verminderte Leistungen bei neuropsychologischen Untersuchungen und Marklager-Veränderungen (Pérez-Dueñas et al. 2005, Moyle et al. 2007, Anderson und Leuzzi 2010).

Adipositas

Unsere Daten bestätigten das Auftreten von Übergewicht bzw. Adipositas bei knapp 40% der adoleszenten und adulten PKU-Patienten. Ein Zusammenhang zwischen Phe-bilanzierter Diät und Adipositas wurde auch in anderen Studien bereits beschrieben, vorwiegend bei PKU-Patienten weiblichen Geschlechts (Acosta et al. 2003, Burrage et al. 2012, White et al. 1982). Dennoch bestätigen unsere wie auch früher erhobene Daten, dass eine Erhöhung des BMI bei PKU-Patienten nicht mit einer erhöhten Gesamtkalorienzufuhr assoziiert sein muss (Acosta 1996). Wir konnten aufzeigen, dass der BMI invers mit der

Zufuhr an Gesamtprotein bzw. synthetischem Protein korreliert. Die unregelmäßig über den Tag verteilte Proteinzufuhr sowie die hohe Kohlenhydratzufuhr der Phe-bilanzierten Diät haben einen Einfluss auf die Ausschüttung von Insulin und auf die Ausschüttung des Appetit-anregenden Hormons Ghrelin, was als eine der möglichen Ursache der Adipositas bei PKU-Patienten postuliert wurde (MacLeod et al. 2010, Weigel et al. 2007).

Arterielle Hypertonie

Anhand unserer Untersuchungen konnten wir erstmals nachweisen, dass PKU-Patienten ein erhöhtes Risiko aufweisen, eine arterielle Hypertonie zu entwickeln (Publikation 2). Bei einem Viertel der adoleszenten und adulten PKU-Patienten wurde eine arterielle Hypertonie diagnostiziert. Zudem fehlte bei über 40% der Patienten der physiologische nächtliche Blutdruckabfall. Das Auftreten einer arteriellen Hypertonie war signifikant mit ansteigendem BMI assoziiert, nicht jedoch mit der Proteinzufuhr, der GFR oder der Proteinausscheidung. Diese Daten weisen darauf hin, dass eine mögliche arterielle Hypertonie bei Patienten mit PKU ein weiteres sekundäres Gesundheitsproblem darstellt. Die Langzeituntersuchungen bei Patienten mit PKU sollten daher unbedingt auch regelmäßige Blutdruck-Kontrollen, insbesondere bei übergewichtigen und adipösen Patienten, beinhalten.

3.1.2. Nierenfunktion bei Patienten mit Phenylalanin-bilanzierter Diät

Wir konnten zudem erstmals nachweisen, dass PKU-Patienten unter der lebenslangen Phe-bilanzierten Diät eine chronische Nierenerkrankung mit eingeschränkter Nierenfunktion, Proteinurie, Mikroalbuminurie und Hyperkalziurie entwickeln können (Publikation 2). Multiple lineare Regressionsanalysen ergaben eine signifikante Assoziation der GFR, gemessen mittels ^{51}Cr-EDTA Isotopen-Clearance, mit der aktuellen Gesamt-Protein-Zufuhr und der Proteinurie. Daraus folgt, dass die Proteinzufuhr und die Proteinurie unabhängig voneinander an dem Pathomechanismus der Nierenschädigung bei Patienten mit PKU beteiligt sind.

Einschränkung der Glomerulären Filtrationsrate

Die GFR, gemessen mittels ^{51}Cr-EDTA Isotopen-Clearance, war signifikant mit steigender Proteinzufuhr assoziiert, sowohl mit der aktuellen als auch mit der lebenslangen Proteinzufuhr, sowohl mit der Zufuhr an Gesamtprotein als auch mit der Zufuhr an synthetischem Protein. 19% der Patienten wiesen eine eingeschränkte GFR auf, lediglich 7% eine Hyperfiltration. Die Proteinzufuhr scheint somit ein wichtiger Risikofaktor in der Genese der chronischen Nierenerkrankung bei Patienten mit PKU zu sein.

Proteinurie

Eine Proteinurie wurde bei über 30% der PKU-Patienten nachgewiesen, eine Mikroalbuminurie bei 7% der Patienten. Unsere Analysen bestätigen, dass die Proteinurie eine unabhängige Variable der Nierenschädigung bei Patienten mit PKU ist. Eine Hyperaminoazidurie fand sich bei keinem Patienten. Die Phe-Ausscheidung im Urin korrelierte jedoch signifikant mit der Proteinurie und der GFR. Dies führte zu der Annahme, dass die erhöhte Phe-Konzentration im Urin einen zusätzlichen Einfluss auf die Nierenschädigung bei Patienten mit PKU haben könnte.

Übergewicht ist ein bekannter Risikofaktor bei der Entwicklung einer Glomerulosklerose (Kambham et al. 2001). Dies entspricht unseren Daten, die eine signifikante Assoziation zwischen BMI und GFR nachwiesen. Dennoch zeigte sich kein Zusammenhang zwischen dem BMI und der Proteinausscheidung. Eine Adipositas scheint somit ein weiterer Risikofaktor für eine chronische Nierenerkrankung bei PKU-Patienten zu sein.

Hyperkalziurie

23% der untersuchten Patienten zeigten ein Hyperkalziurie. Die Kalziumausscheidung stieg mit steigender Proteinzufuhr signifikant an, vor allem mit steigender Zufuhr an synthetischem Protein, wobei die lebenslange Proteinzufuhr keinen Einfluss auf die Kalziumausscheidung hatte. Eine mögliche Hyperkalziurie birgt somit ein weiteres Langzeitrisiko für PKU-Patienten. Dennoch war die Hyperkalziurie nicht mit verminderter GFR, Proteinurie oder arterieller Hypertonie assoziiert, und nur wenige Patienten wiesen eine Nephrokalzinose auf. Eine Assoziation mit den Serumkonzentrationen von 25-Hydroxy-Vitamin D(3) oder 1,25-Dihydroxy-Vitamin D(3) bestand ebenfalls nicht. Obwohl die aktuellen Empfehlungen zur Nährstoffzufuhr eine höhere Vitamin D-Zufuhr bei Adoleszenten und Erwachsenen anraten (German Nutrition Society 2012), wies keiner der hier untersuchten PKU-Patienten einen Vitamin D-Mangel auf.

3.1.3. Genese der Nierenschädigung unter Phenylalanin-bilanzierter Diät

Mehrere Pathomechanismen können als Ursache der renalen Schädigung bei Patienten mit PKU in Erwägung gezogen werden:

1. Ein Zusammenhang zwischen der diätetischen Proteinzufuhr und der Nierenfunktion ist seit langem bekannt (Brenner et al. 1982; King und Levey 1993). Die Hyperfiltrationstheorie besagt, dass eine hohe Proteinzufuhr zu einem akuten Anstieg des renalen Plasmaflusses und der GFR führt, resultierend in Hyperfiltration, glomerulärer Schädigung und chronischer Niereninsuffizienz (Bernstein et al. 2007; Brenner et al. 1996). Daher wird bei Patienten mit

terminaler Niereninsuffizienz eine protein-restriktive Kost empfohlen (Brenner et al 1982; Fouque und Aparicio 2007). Die Gesamt-Proteinzufuhr bei PKU-Patienten übersteigt häufig die geltenden Diät-Empfehlungen (MacDonald et al. 2011), und auch in unserem Patientenkollektiv wurde die empfohlene Gesamt-Proteinzufuhr deutlich überschritten. Dennoch lag die Gesamt-Proteinzufuhr der untersuchten PKU-Patienten noch in dem Bereich einer „normalen" westlichen Ernährung, weshalb die Gesamt-Proteinzufuhr als alleiniger Faktor eine chronische Nierenerkrankung bei Patienten mit PKU nicht hinreichend erklärt (Fouque und Aparicio 2007; Halbesma et al. 2009).

2. Die Proteinzufuhr bei PKU-Patienten unterscheidet sich jedoch in ihrer Zusammensetzung deutlich von der Proteinzufuhr Gesunder und besteht zu mehr als Zweidritteln aus dem synthetischen Aminosäurengemisch. Nach Zufuhr des aus Mono-Aminosäuren bestehenden Aminosäurengemisches zeigen sich hohe Plasma-Aminosäuren-Peaks (Gropper et al. 1993, Mönch et al. 1996). Im Tiermodell waren hohe Plasma-Aminosäuren-Spiegel nephrotoxisch und führten zu einem signifikanten Abfall der GFR mit Albuminurie und histologisch nachweisbarer tubulärer Schädigung (Zager et al. 1983). Ein ähnlicher Pathomechanismus könnte demnach ursächlich für die Nierenschädigungen bei Patienten mit PKU sein.

Zudem konnte in Studien ein Einfluss des synthetischen Aminosäurengemisches auf die Steigerung des Blut-Harnstoff-Stickstoffs und die Harnstoff-Synthese nachgewiesen werden (van Calcar et al. 2009). Im Mausmodell resultierte nach der Zufuhr von Aminosäurengemischen eine Zunahme der Nierenmasse, wahrscheinlich bedingt durch eine erhöhte renale Auslastung, um den nach Aminosäuren-Zufuhr anfallenden Harnstoff besser eliminieren zu können (Solverson et al. 2012).

3. Die Ausscheidung von Phe im Urin war signifikant mit der GFR und der Proteinurie assoziiert. Obwohl bislang kein nephrotoxischer Effekt von Phe bekannt ist, kann nicht ausgeschlossen werden, dass hohe Phe-Konzentrationen im Urin einen zusätzlichen Einfluss auf die Entwicklung der chronischen Nierenerkrankung bei Patienten mit PKU haben.

4. Erhöhter oxidativer Stress ist bei Patienten mit PKU mehrfach nachgewiesen worden. Ursache hierfür sind die erhöhte Bildung freier Radikale, ein potentieller Mangel an Mikronährstoffen sowie ein Anstieg von Phe und dessen Metaboliten (Ribas et al. 2011). Erhöhter oxidativer Stress könnte eine entscheidende Rolle in der Pathogenese der renalen Gewebeschädigung und der chronischen Nierenerkrankung bei PKU spielen.

5. Es wurde beschrieben, dass die menschliche Niere eine wichtige Funktion in der Phe-Homöostase einnimmt. PAH wird nicht nur in der Leber sondern auch in der menschlichen Niere exprimiert (Lichter- Konecki et al. 1999), und eine Verminderung der PAH-Aktivität ist

bei Niereninsuffizienz bekannt (Zhao et al. 2012). Die renale *PAH*-Expression könnte daher einen Einfluss auf die Nierenfunktion ausüben, obwohl unsere Daten keinen Zusammenhang zwischen der chronischen Nierenerkrankung und dem *PAH*-Genotyp aufzeigen.

Anhand dieser Daten wird jedoch deutlich, dass bei adoleszenten und adulten Patienten unter einer Phe-bilanzierten Diät regelmäßige Untersuchungen der Nierenfunktion unbedingt durchgeführt sollten.

3.2. Therapie mit Tetrahydrobiopterin

Mit der Erstbeschreibung der BH4-responsiven PKU im Jahr 1999 (Kure et al. 1999) avancierte BH4 zur möglichen Alternative in der Behandlung von Patienten mit PKU. Zunächst war BH4 in Deutschland über Schircks Laboratories (Schweiz) erhältlich. Sapropterin-Dihydrochlorid (Kuvan®; Merck Serono SA, Schweiz), eine synthetisch hergestellte Form von BH4, erhielt 2007 die Zulassung durch die *Food and Drug Administration* in den U.S.A. und 2009 die Zulassung durch die Europäische Arzneimittel-Agentur EMEA in Deutschland (Burnett 2007, Ziesch et al. 2012). Beide BH4-Produkte enthalten die gleiche aktive Substanz 6R-BH4 (Burnett 2007). Die Einführung von BH4 als neue therapeutische Option bei Patienten mit PKU wurde mit großem Optimismus und Enthusiasmus aufgenommen. Es wurde geschätzt, dass mindestens 30% der Patienten mit PKU von einer BH4-Behandlung profitieren könnten (Bernegger und Blau 2002, Zurflüh et al. 2006).

Verschiedene Ursachen für die Wirkung von BH4 bei Patienten mit einer BH4-responsiven PKU wurden diskutiert, wie z. B. Mutationen im Bereich der BH4-bindenden Domäne der PAH, mögliche K_m-Varianten der PAH, eine verminderte Bindung von BH4 an die mutierte PAH oder suboptimale physiologische BH4-Konzentrationen (Aguado et al. 2007, Erlandsen und Stevens 2001, Kure et al. 2004). Inzwischen wird die These des pharmakologischen Chaperoneffekts von BH4 favorisiert. Danach fungiert BH4 in pharmakologisch hohen Dosen als Chaperon und führt zu einer Stabilisierung des mutierten Enzyms, zu einer Verhinderung des Enzymabbaus sowie zu einer Verminderung von Enzymaggregation, was in einer Erhöhung der PAH-Restenzymaktivität resultiert (Muntau und Gersting 2010).

3.2.1. Identifikation von langzeit-BH4-responsiven PKU-Patienten

Eine Langzeittherapie mit BH4 ist mittlerweile bei einigen größeren Patientengruppen mit BH4-responsiver PKU berichtet worden (Burton et al. 2007, Lee et al. 2008, Levy et al. 2007, Trefz et al. 2010). Die meisten dieser Studien konzentrierten sich vorwiegend auf den Effekt von BH4 auf eine Reduktion der Phe-Blutwerte (Burton et al. 2007, Lee et al. 2008, Levy et al. 2007) und nicht auf eine Steigerung der individuellen Phe-Toleranz. In unseren Studien konnten wir jedoch beide Effekte einer BH4-Therapie nachweisen (Publikation 3, Publikation 4, Publikation 6).

Die Steigerung der Phe-Toleranz unter der BH4-Therapie ist für die Patienten von großer Bedeutung, da dies eine größere Freiheit in der Diätführung und eine deutliche Verbesserung der Lebensqualität impliziert. Gleichwohl gestaltet sich die Identifikation von Patienten mit einer BH4-responsiven PKU, insbesondere solcher Patienten, die auf eine Langzeittherapie mit BH4 ansprechen, weiterhin als schwierig. Kriterien zur Identifikation langzeit-BH4-responsiver PKU-Patienten existierten bislang nicht. Uns gelang es erstmals, Kriterien festzulegen, mit denen bereits in der Neonatalperiode potentiell BH4-responsive PKU-Patienten identifiziert werden können (Publikation 6).

BH4-Belastungstest

Ursprünglich wurde der BH4-Belastungstest zur Diagnose von Patienten mit einem Defekt in der Synthese bzw. Regeneration von BH4 etabliert. Diese Patienten zeigen im BH4-Belastungstest bereits 3-7 Stunden nach BH4-Gabe einen Abfall der Phe-Werte (Curtius et al. 1979, Ponzone et al. 1993). Patienten mit einer BH4-responsiven PKU dagegen weisen im BH4-Belastungstest erst >8 Stunden nach BH4-Gabe einen Abfall der Phe-Werte auf (Kure et al. 1999, Zurflüh et al. 2006). Der BH4-Test wird als positiv gewertet, wenn ein Abfall von mindestens 30% des basalen Phe-Wertes erreicht wird (Bernegger und Blau 2002). In der Praxis werden zur Identifikation von Patienten mit einer BH4-responsiven PKU unterschiedliche BH4-Belastungstests benutzt (Blau et al. 2010). All diese BH4-Belastungstests können jedoch sowohl falsch negative wie auch falsch positive Ergebnisse erbringen, beispielsweise bedingt durch ein verzögertes Ansprechen auf BH4, eine zu niedrige BH4-Dosis, eine zu niedrige Phe-Zufuhr, mangelnde Compliance oder eine katabole Stoffwechselsituation (Blau et al. 2009, Nielsen et al. 2010, Publikation 7). Ein Großteil dieser Störfaktoren scheint im Neugeborenenalter eine weniger bedeutende Rolle zu spielen als in späterem Lebensalter.

In Europa wird derzeit der BH4-Belastungstest bei mindestens der Hälfte der Neugeborenen, die im Neonatalscreening mit einer Phe-Erhöhung von >400 µmol/L diagnostiziert werden, durchgeführt (Blau et al. 2010). Wir konnten anhand unserer Daten nachweisen, dass der neonatale BH4-Belastungstest über 24 Stunden ein guter prädiktiver Faktor ist, um eine potentielle Langzeit-BH4-Responsivität vorherzusagen. Dennoch können PKU-Patienten, die eine verzögerte BH4-Responsivität aufweisen, sogenannte "*slow responder*", mit dem BH4-Belastungstest über einen Zeitraum von nur 24 Stunden nicht sicher erfasst werden. Daher muss, zumindest in Einzelfällen, eine Verlängerung des BH4-Belastungstests bis mindestens 48 Stunden in Erwägung gezogen werden (Fiege et al. 2005). Ein positiver BH4-Belastungstest sagt allerdings nicht sicher eine Langzeit-BH4-Responsivität vorher wie auch ein negativer BH4-Belastungstest eine Langzeit-BH4-Responsivität nicht sicher ausschließt.

Identifikation mittels Phänotyps

Wir konnten anhand unserer Daten nachweisen, dass nicht nur Patienten mit einem milden PKU-Phänotyp BH4-responsiv sein können sondern auch Patienten mit einem schweren PKU-Phänotyp (Publikation 3). Auch bei diesen Patienten kann durch die BH4-Therapie sowohl ein Abfall der Phe-Blutwerte als auch eine Steigerung der individuellen Phe-Toleranz erreicht werden.

Langzeit-BH4-Responder können auch anhand klinischer Daten identifiziert werden. Hierzu zählen insbesondere die maximalen Phe-Blutspiegel und die maximale Phe/Tyr-Ratio, sowohl bei Diagnosestellung als auch unter diätetischer Therapie. Die Phe-Toleranz allein scheint kein sicheres Identifikationsmerkmal darzustellen. Dies ist vermutlich dadurch bedingt, dass die durch unsere Studien ermittelte Phe-Toleranz mittels ambulanter Kontrollen zu Hause bestimmt wurde, was potentiell fehlerbelasteter ist als eine standardisierte Bestimmung unter stationären Bedingungen.

Identifikation mittels Genotyps

Derzeit sind mehr als 700 verschiedene *PAH*-Mutationen bekannt, und mehr als 400 verschiedene Mutationskombinationen wurden bislang bei Patienten mit einer BH4-responsiven PKU beschrieben (*http://www.biopku.org/biopku*). Meist betrifft dies „mildere" Mutationen, die mit einer höheren PAH-Restaktivität assoziiert sind. Sogenannte Nullmutationen mit nur geringer PAH-Restaktivität sind nicht mit einer BH4-Responsivität assoziiert (*http://www.biopku.org/biopku*). Obwohl wir auch bei einigen Patienten mit einem schweren PKU-Phänotyp eine BH4-Responsivität nachweisen konnten, waren alle diese Patienten Träger zumindest einer milderen oder varianten *PAH*-Mutation (Publikation 3, Publikation 7).

Dennoch zeigen auch unsere Daten, dass der Genotyp allein keine zuverlässige Aussage über eine potentielle Langzeit-BH4-Responsivität liefert. Bei einigen Genotypen, z. B. bei der Kombination mit den *PAH*-Mutationen p.Y414C, p.A403V, p.A300S und p.R261, ist eine BH4-Responsivität sicher zu erwarten, bei einigen anderen Mutationen dagegen nicht immer. Einen Erklärungsansatz hierfür liefert die These der sogenannten interallelischen Komplementation. Von einer interallelischen Komplementation spricht man, wenn Mutationen in Compound-Heterozygotie vorliegen und das daraus resultierende Genprodukt weniger oder mehr aktiv ist als das Genprodukt der Mutationen in homozygotem Zustand (Leandro et al. 2011). Dies ist von besonderer Bedeutung bei Erkrankungen, die eine hohe Rate an compound-heterozygoten Genotypen aufweisen. Für die PKU trifft dies in besonderem Maße zu, da bis zu 75% der Patienten einen compound-heterozygoten Genotyp aufweisen (Publikation 1, Leandro et al. 2011). Kürzlich wurde außerdem nachgewiesen, dass variante *PAH*-Mutationen abhängig von ihrer zweiten Mutation *in trans* unterschiedlich auf BH4 reagieren. Ein Beispiel hierfür bietet die Missense-Mutation p.R261Q: In homozygotem Zustand ist diese Mutation mit einer BH4-Responsivität assoziiert, in Heterozygotie mit einer Nullmutation dagegen nicht (Staudigl et al. 2011). Dies wird ebenfalls durch unsere Untersuchungen bestätigt, in denen wir eine Langzeit-BH4-Responsivität bei Patienten mit Homozygotie für p.R261Q nachweisen konnten, bei Patienten mit einer Compound-Hetereozygotie für p.R261Q allerdings nicht.

Auch wenn die molekulargenetische Analyse des *PAH*-Gens bei der PKU keinen diagnostischen Stellenwert besitzt, so konnten auch wir anhand unserer Daten aufzeigen, dass die Aussagekraft dieser Analyse gerade für eine mögliche Therapieoption mit BH4 von großer Bedeutung ist (Publikation 7).

3.2.2. Prädiktive Parameter für Langzeit-BH4-Responsivität

Unsere Daten zeigen, dass es keinen einzelnen spezifischen Parameter gibt, der eine Langzeit-BH4-Responsivität vorhersagt. Durch die Analyse bestimmter laborchemischer, molekulargenetischer und klinischer Daten ist jedoch eine sichere Einschätzung über eine potentielle Langzeit-BH4-Responsivität möglich. Die Kombination folgender Parameter erlaubt bereits bei der Diagnosestellung im Neugeborenenalter eine Aussage über eine potentielle BH4-Responsivität: maximale Phe-Konzentration bei Diagnosestellung <1200 μmol/L, maximale Phe/Tyr-Ratio bei Diagnosestellung <15, positiver neonataler BH4-Belastungstest und mindestens eine potentiell BH4-responsive Mutation. Dies ermöglicht eine frühe Einschätzung über mögliche Therapieoptionen und eine entsprechende Beratung der betroffenen Familien.

Zudem gibt es mehrere Faktoren, die eine Langzeit-BH4-Responsivität beeinflussen, wie in besonderem Maße die jeweilige Stoffwechseleinstellung. Eine Langzeittherapie mit BH4 scheint sowohl die Stabilität von PAH als auch den Chaperoneffekt von BH4 zu stärken (Staudigl et al. 2011). Auch aus diesem Grund empfehlen wir eine verlängerte Testung von BH4 bei potentiell langzeit-BH4-responsiven PKU-Patienten. Unsere Daten zeigen überdies, dass einige Patienten nur langsam ihre individuelle Phe-Toleranz steigern können, so dass der Effekt einer BH4-Langzeittherapie erst im Verlauf von mindestens drei Monaten nach Beginn der BH4-Behandlung erkannt werden kann.

Die Annahme, dass 30% der Patienten mit PKU von einer BH4-Behandlung profitieren könnten (Bernegger und Blau 2002, Zurflüh et al. 2006), wurde durch unsere Daten nicht belegt. In unserem Patientenkollektiv lag das Langzeit-Ansprechen auf BH4 bei nur 15%. Möglicherweise ist dies durch unser Patientenkollektiv bestimmt, das eine hohe Rate an Patienten mit einer klassischen PKU und eine hohe Rate an Nullmutationen, insbesondere der Punktmutation p.R408W, aufwies (Publikation 1).

3.2.3. Langzeittherapie mit Tetrahydrobiopterin

Diätumstellung unter BH4-Langzeittherapie

Der Beginn einer Langzeittherapie mit BH4 erfordert strenge Kontrollen der Phe-Blutwerte sowie der Phe-Zufuhr. Dies ist nur bei guter Zusammenarbeit mit den betroffenen Patienten und deren Eltern möglich. Wir etablierten eine effektive Methode, mit der nach einem Stufenplan schrittweise die Phe-Zufuhr gesteigert, die eiweißarmen Lebensmittel durch normale Produkte ersetzt und das Aminosäurengemisch reduziert werden können (Publikation 6). Dieser Stufenplan wurde von den Patienten und deren Eltern sehr gut akzeptiert, obwohl sie der Diätlockerung zunächst mit Angst und großer Vorsicht begegneten. Die Patienten mit PKU, die zuvor ausschließlich eine Phe-bilanzierte Diät erhielten, entwickelten nach Lockerung der Diät unter BH4 besondere Essgewohnheiten. Viele PKU-Patienten lehnten eiweißreiche Lebensmittel ab, insbesondere Kuhmilch, Milchprodukte und Fisch. Ein Großteil der Patienten, die unter der BH4-Therapie ihre Phe-bilanzierte Diät beenden konnten, benötigte weiterhin eine Supplementation mit Vitaminen und Mikronährstoffen. Die Gefahr einer Mikronährstoff-Defizienz wurde durch andere Studien bestätigt (Singh et al. 2010). Unter der Langzeittherapie mit BH4 ist es daher erforderlich, die diätetische Zufuhr und die Serumspiegel bestimmter Mikronährstoffe und Vitamine zu kontrollieren, v. a. die von Kalzium, Eisen, Vitamin B12 und Vitamin D. Dies betrifft vorwiegend Patienten mit PKU, die unter der BH4-Langzeittherapie kein Aminosäurengemisch mehr erhalten.

Wie wir in unseren Studien nachweisen konnten, wurde die Lockerung der Phe-bilanzierten Diät unter der Behandlung mit BH4 sowohl von den Patienten als auch von deren Eltern als eine deutliche Steigerung ihrer Lebensqualität empfunden. Die Lebensqualität wurde in unseren Untersuchungen ausschließlich anamnestisch befragt. Im Gegensatz hierzu wurde in einer kürzlich durchgeführten Studie keine Steigerung der gesundheitsbezogenen Lebensqualität unter der Behandlung mit BH4 berichtet (Ziesch et al. 2012).

Dosierung von BH4

Dosierungen von BH4 sind in der Literatur mit 5-20 mg/kg KG/die beschrieben (Lee et al. 2008, Levy et al. 2007). Dennoch benötigten die meisten der von uns untersuchten Patienten höhere BH4-Dosen von mindestens 15 mg/kg KG/die, insbesondere Patienten mit einem schweren PKU-Phänotyp, die unter BH4-Therapie weiterhin ein Aminosäurengemisch einnahmen. Niedrigere BH4-Dosierungen waren lediglich bei einigen wenigen Patienten mit einem milden PKU-Phänotyp effektiv. Dies wurde durch eine kürzlich publizierte Arbeit bestätigt (Staudigl et al. 2011). Wir konnten zudem aufzeigen, dass durch eine Titrierung der individuellen BH4-Dosis eine stufenweise Reduktion der BH4-Dosis erreicht werden kann. Bei Beginn einer BH4-Therapie sollte die initiale Dosis von BH4 bei 20 mg/kg KG/die liegen und individuell nach den Phe-Blutwerten sowie der Phe-Toleranz adaptiert werden.

Nebenwirkungen der BH4-Therapie

In unseren (Publikation 4, Publikation 5) und anderen BH4-Langzeitstudien (Lee et al. 2008, Levy et al. 2007) traten einige unerwünschte Ereignisse wie gastrointestinale Probleme, Rhinorrhoe und Kopfschmerzen auf, die als möglicherweise medikamentenassoziierte Nebenwirkungen von BH4 einzustufen sind. Die gastrointestinalen Probleme unter BH4-Therapie könnten möglicherweise durch den säurehaltigen Charakter des Produktes bedingt sein. Wir konnten außerdem nachweisen, dass einige Patienten unter der BH4-Therapie eine intermittierende Transaminasenerhöhung, eine transiente Neutropenie oder Thrombozytopenie aufweisen. Auch diese Laborveränderungen sind als möglicherweise medikamentenassoziiert einzustufen. Bei einigen wenigen Patienten zeigte sich unter der BH4-Therapie eine kurzzeitige Erniedrigung der Phe-Blutkonzentration auf Werte <26 µmol/L. Unter der Langzeittherapie mit BH4 sollten daher neben regelmäßigen Kontrollen der Phe-Blutwerte auch regelmäßige Kontrollen der Transaminasen sowie des Blutbildes inklusive Differenzierung erfolgen. Geschmack und Konsistenz von BH4 wurde von einigen Patienten in unserem Patientenkollektiv als sehr unangenehm empfunden; gleichwohl beendete keiner der Patienten die BH4-Therapie aufgrund dieser Unverträglichkeiten.

Indikation für eine BH4-Langzeittherapie

Trotz des positiven Effekts von BH4 auf eine Steigerung der individuellen Phe-Toleranz und auf eine Reduktion der Phe-Blutwerte ist die Indikation zu einer Langzeittherapie mit BH4 nach unseren Ergebnissen streng zu stellen. Insbesondere Patienten mit einer milden PKU profitieren von der BH4-Therapie, während Patienten mit einem schweren PKU-Phänotyp zwar BH4-responsiv sein können, aber unter der Langzeittherapie mit BH4 meist nur eine geringe Steigerung ihrer Phe-Toleranz erreichen. Für eine BH4-Langzeittherapie setzten wir eine mindestens 2,5fache Steigerung der initialen Phe-Toleranz voraus. Dies entspricht auch Daten aus anderen Studien (Singh et al. 2010). Bei der Entscheidung über eine BH4-Langzeittherapie ist zudem der Kostenfaktor zu berücksichtigen. Die von uns kalkulierten Kosten für eine BH4-Therapie in einer Dosis von 10 mg/kg KG/die betragen bereits im Alter von 6 Monaten das 1,5-fache der Phe-bilanzierten Diät inkl. des Aminosäurengemisches, ab dem zweiten Lebensjahr sogar das 2-fache. Bei BH4-Dosierungen von 20 mg/kg KG/die liegen die Kosten dementsprechend zwischen 3- bis 4-fach höher als unter der herkömmlichen diätetischen Therapie.

3.3. Ausblick

BH4 ist nicht nur Kofaktor aromatischer Hydroxylasen sondern auch Kofaktor der Nitritoxid-Synthase. Die Nitritoxid-Synthase und somit auch BH4 nehmen eine zentrale Rolle in der Regulation der vaskulären Homöostase ein. Eine Depletion von BH4 führt zu endothelialer Dysfunktion, verstärkter Gefäßinflammation sowie der Zunahme arteriosklerotischer Veränderungen und folglich zu kardiovaskulären Erkrankungen (Alkaitis und Crabtree 2012, McNeill und Channon 2012). Der therapeutische Effekt von BH4 auf kardiovaskuläre Erkrankungen wird derzeit in mehreren Studien untersucht. Eine Pilotstudie konnte einen antihypertensiven Effekt von BH4 bei Patienten mit schlecht eingestellter arterieller Hypertonie nachweisen (Porkert et al. 2008), während eine kürzlich veröffentlichte Studie keinen Effekt einer BH4-Therapie auf die Gefäßfunktion und den Redoxstatus von Patienten mit einer koronaren Gefäßerkrankung aufzeigte (Cunnington et al. 2012).

Wie in dieser Arbeit dargestellt, weisen Patienten mit PKU ein erhöhtes Risiko auf, eine arterielle Hypertonie oder eine chronische Nierenerkrankung zu entwickeln. Zudem ist bei Patienten mit PKU erhöhter oxidativer Stress mit vermehrter Bildung freier Radikale beschrieben (Ribas et al. 2011). Die arterielle Hypertonie, die chronische Nierenerkrankung und der erhöhte oxidative Stress bei PKU-Patienten könnten auch durch einen relativen BH4-Mangel bedingt sein. In diesem Zusammenhang könnte BH4 eine zusätzliche Therapieoption bei PKU-Patienten mit arterieller Hypertonie oder chronischer Nierenerkrankung darstellen.

4. Zusammenfassung

Trotz Etablierung neuer Therapieoptionen ist die Phe-bilanzierte Diät weiterhin die Therapie der Wahl bei Patienten mit einer PKU, insbesondere bei Patienten mit einer klassischen PKU. Bekannte Langzeitprobleme bei Patienten mit PKU sind neurologische Defizite, Mikronährstoff-Defizite, Osteopenie und Adipositas. Wie in dieser Arbeit dargestellt, weisen PKU-Patienten unter der Phe-bilanzierten Diät zudem ein erhöhtes Risiko auf, eine arterielle Hypertonie sowie eine chronische Nierenerkrankung mit eingeschränkter Nierenfunktion, Proteinurie, Mikroalbuminurie und Hyperkalziurie zu entwickeln. Mögliche Ursachen der chronischen Nierenerkrankung bei PKU-Patienten sind die hohe Gesamteiweißzufuhr, die hohe Zufuhr von Mono-Aminosäuren über das Aminosäurengemisch, lokale Schädigungen durch die hohe Phe-Ausscheidung sowie erhöhter oxidativer Stress.

Die Therapie mit BH4, dem Kofaktor der PAH, stellt eine alternative Behandlungsoption für einige Patienten mit PKU dar. Das Ansprechen auf BH4 wird bestimmt durch den Genotyp und den daraus resultierenden Phänotyp. Populationen mit einer hohen Rate an Nullmutationen weisen eine geringere Rate an BH4-responsiven PKU-Patienten auf. Anhand unserer Daten konnten wir nachweisen, dass durch die Analyse bestimmter laborchemischer, molekulargenetischer und klinischer Daten bereits in der Neonatalperiode eine Einschätzung über eine potentielle Langzeit-BH4-Responsivität möglich ist.

Bei BH4-responsiven PKU-Patienten führt die Therapie mit BH4 zu einer Reduzierung der Phe-Blutwerte und zu einer Steigerung der individuellen Phe-Toleranz. Die Langzeittherapie mit BH4 sollte nach einem klar definierten Protokoll durchgeführt werden, insbesondere bezüglich der Steigerung der individuellen Phe-Toleranz und der BH4-Dosierung. Gleichwohl muss die Indikation zu einer BH4-Langzeittherapie kritisch gestellt werden. Vorwiegend Patienten mit einer milden PKU profitieren von der BH4-Therapie, während Patienten mit einem schweren PKU-Phänotyp zwar BH4-responsiv sein können, aber unter der Langzeittherapie mit BH4 meist nur eine geringe Steigerung ihrer Phe-Toleranz erreichen. Für eine BH4-Langzeittherapie ist eine mindestens 2,5-fache Steigerung der initialen Phe-Toleranz vorauszusetzen. Die Kosten einer Therapie mit BH4 liegen zwischen 1,5- bis 4-fach höher als die der Phe-bilanzierten Diät. Mögliche Nebenwirkungen der BH4-Langzeittherapie können gastrointestinale Probleme, Kopfschmerzen und Mikronährstoff-Defizite sein.

Dennoch ist die Bedeutung von BH4 in der Behandlung der PKU nicht zu unterschätzen. BH4 nimmt als Kofaktor der Nitroxid-Synthase eine Schlüsselfunktion in der Regulation der vaskulären Homöostase ein, weshalb eine Depletion von BH4 in der Pathogenese kardiovaskulärer Erkrankungen eine entscheidende Rolle spielt. Ein relativer BH4-Mangel könnte somit bei PKU-Patienten einen Einfluss auf den erhöhten oxidativen Stress, die arterielle Hypertonie und die chronische Nierenerkrankung haben. In diesem Zusammenhang könnte BH4 eine zusätzliche Bedeutung in der Behandlung von PKU-Patienten einnehmen. Andere neue Therapieoptionen werden derzeit sowohl in klinischen Studien als auch in Tiermodellen untersucht, und sie könnten in Zukunft eine mögliche Alternative zu der Phe-bilanzierten Diät darstellen.

5. Literaturangaben aus dem freien Text

Acosta PB, Yannicelli S, Singh R, et al. Nutrient intakes and physical growth of children with phenylketonuria undergoing nutrition therapy. J Am Diet Assoc. 2003;103:1167-1173.

Acosta PB. Recommendations for protein and energy intakes by patients with phenylketonuria. Eur J Pediatr. 1996;155 Suppl 1:S121–S124.

Aguado C, Pérez B, García MJ, et al. BH4 responsiveness associated to a PKU mutation with decreased binding affinity for the cofactor. Clin Chim Acta. 2007;380:8-12.

Ahring KK. Large neutral amino acids in daily practice. Inherit Metab Dis. 2010;DOI: 10.1007/s10545-010-9069-7.

Alkaitis MS, Crabtree MJ. Recoupling the Cardiac Nitric Oxide Synthases: Tetrahydrobiopterin Synthesis and Recycling. Curr Heart Fail Rep. 2012;9:200–210.

Anderson PJ, Leuzzi V. White matter pathology in phenylketonuria. Mol Genet Metab. 2010;99 Suppl 1:S3-S9.

BAnz. Bekanntmachung des Bundesministeriums für Gesundheit und soziale Sicherung. Kinder-Richtlinien. Nr. 60 (S. 4833) vom 31.03.2005

Bauman ML, Kemper TL. Morphologic and histoanatomic observations of the brain in untreated human phenylketonuria. Acta Neuropathol. 1982;58:55-63.

Bernegger C, Blau N. High frequency of tetrahydrobiopterin-responsiveness among hyperphenylalaninemias: a study of 1,919 patients observed from 1988 to 2002. Mol Genet Metab. 2002;77:304-313.

Bernstein AM, Treyzon L, Li Z. Are high-protein, vegetable based diets safe for kidney function? A review of the literature. J Am Diet Assoc. 2007;107:644-650.

Bickel H, Gerrard J, Hickmans EM. Influence of phenylalanine intake on phenylketonuria. Lancet. 1953;265:812-813.

Binek-Singer P, Johnson TC. The effects of chronic hyperphenylalaninaemia on mouse brain protein synthesis can be prevented by other amino acids. Biochem J. 1982;206:407-414.

Blau N, Bélanger-Quintana A, Demirkol M, et al. Optimizing the use of Sapropterin (BH(4)) in the management of phenylketonuria. Mol Genet Metab. 2009;96:158-163.

Blau N, Belanger-Quintana A, Demirkol M, et al. Management of phenylketonuria in Europe: Survey results from 19 countries. Mol Genet Metab. 2010;99:109-115.

Boado RJ, Li JY, Nagaya M, Zhang C, Pardridge WM. Selective expression of the large neutral amino acid transporter at the blood-brain barrier. Proc Natl Acad Sci USA. 1999;96:12079-12084.

Böhles H, Hoffmann G, Kohlmüller D, Mayatepek E, Sewell A, Wagner L. Befunde des metabolischen Labors. Darstellung typischer Laborbefunde bei der Diagnostik angeborener Stoffwechselerkrankungen. 1999. SHS Ges. für Klinische Ernährung mbH, Heilbronn.

Brenner BM, Lawler EV, Mackenzie HS. The hyperfiltration theory: a paradigm shift in nephrology. Kidney Int. 1996;49:1774-1777.

Brenner BM, Meyer TW, Hostetter TH. Dietary protein intake and the progressive nature of kidney disease. N Engl J Med. 1982;307:652-659.

Burgard P, Bremer HJ, Bührdel P, et al. Rationale for the German recommendations for phenylalanine level control in phenylketonuria 1997. Eur J Pediat. 1999;158:46-54.

Burlina AB, Bonafé L, Ferrari V, Suppiej A, Zacchello F, Burlina AP. Measurement of neurotransmitter metabolites in the cerebrospinal fluid of phenylketonuric patients under dietary treatment. J Inherit Metab Dis. 2000;23:313-316.

Burnett J. Sapropterin dihydrochloride (Kuvan/phenoptin), an orally active synthetic form of BH4 for the treatment of phenylketonuria. IDrugs. 2007;10:805-13.

Burrage LC, McConnell J, Haesler R, et al. High prevalence of overweight and obesity in females with phenylketonuria. Mol Genet Metab. 2012;107:43-48.

Burton BK, Grange DK, Milanowski A, et al. The response of patients with phenylketonuria and elevated serum phenylalanine to treatment with oral sapropterin dihydrochloride (6R-tetrahydrobiopterin): a phase II, multicentre, open-label, screening study. J Inherit Metab Dis. 2007;30:700-707.

Butler IJ, O'Flynn ME, Seifert WE Jr, Howell RR. Neurotransmitter defects and treatment of disorders of hyperphenylalaninemia. J Pediatr. 1981;98:729-733.

Choi TB, Pardridge WM. Phenylalanine transport at the human blood-brain barrier. Studies with isolated human brain capillaries. J Biol Chem. 1986;261:6536-6541.

Clayton BE, Jenkins P, Round JM. Paediatric Chemical Pathology: Clinical Tests and Reference Ranges. Oxford, Blackwell Scientific Publications, 1980.

Cotugno G, Nicolò R, Cappelletti S, Goffredo BM, Dionisi Vici C, Di Ciommo V. Adherence to diet and quality of life in patients with phenylketonuria. Acta Paediatr. 2011;100:1144-1149.

Cunnington C, Van Assche T, Shirodaria C, et al. Systemic and vascular oxidation limits efficacy of oral tetrahydrobiopterin treatment in patients with coronary artery disease. Circulation. 2012;125:1356-1366.

Curtius HC, Niederwieser A, Viscontini M, et al. Atypical phenylketonuria due to tetrahydrobiopterin deficiency. Diagnosis and treatment with tetrahydrobiopterin, dihydrobiopterin and sepiapterin. Clin Chim Acta. 1979;93:251-262.

D-A-CH Empfehlung: Deutsche Gesellschaft für Ernährung, Österreichische Gesellschaft für Ernährung, Schweizerische Gesellschaft für Ernährungsforschung, Schweizerische Vereinigung für Ernährung. 2000. Referenzwerte für die Nährstoffzufuhr: Umschau/Braus Verlag.

de Groot MJ, Hoeksma M, Blau N, Reijngoud DJ, van Spronsen FJ. Pathogenesis of cognitive dysfunction in phenylketonuria: review of hypotheses. Mol Genet Metab. 2010;99 Suppl 1:S86-S89.

DGE Empfehlung: Deutsche Gesellschaft für Ernährung. 1985. Empfehlungen für die Nährstoffzufuhr: Umschau Verlag.

DiLella AG, Kwok SC, Ledley FD, Marvit J, Woo SL. Molecular structure and polymorphic map of the human phenylalanine hydroxylase gene. Biochemistry. 1986;25:743-749.

Eisensmith RC, Goltsov AA, O'Neill CO, et al. Recurrence of the R408W mutation in the phenylalanine hydroxylase locus in Europeans. Am J Hum Genet. 1995;56:278-286.

Erlandsen H, Stevens RC. A structural hypothesis for BH4 responsiveness in patients with mild forms of hyperphenylalaninemia and phenylketonuria. J Inherit Metab Dis. 2001;24:213-230.

Erlandsen H, Stevens RC. The structural basis of phenylketonuria. Mol Genet Metab. 1999;68:103-125.

Fiege B, Bonafé L, Ballhausen D, et al. Extended tetrahydrobiopterin loading test in the diagnosis of cofactor-responsive phenylketonuria: a pilot study. Mol Genet Metab. 2005;86 Suppl 1:S91-S95.

Følling A. Über Ausscheidung von Phenylbrenztraubensäure in den Harn als Stoffwechselanomalie in Verbindung mit Imbezillität. Hoppe-Seyler's Z Physiol Chem. 1934;227:169-176.

Fouque D, Aparicio M. Eleven reasons to control the protein intake of patients with chronic kidney disease. Nat Clin Pract Nephrol. 2007;3:383-392.

Gámez A, Sarkissian CN, Wang L, et al. Development of pegylated forms of recombinant Rhodosporidium toruloides phenylalanine ammonia-lyase for the treatment of classical phenylketonuria. Mol Ther. 2005;11:986-989.

German Nutrition Society. New reference values for vitamin D. Ann Nutr Metab. 2012;60:241-246.

Gropper SS, Gropper DM, Acosta PB. Plasma amino acid response to ingestion of L-amino acids and whole protein. J Pediatr Gastroenterol Nutr. 1993;16:143-150.

Guldberg P, Rey F, Zschocke J, et al. A European Multicenter Study of Phenylalanine Hydroxylase Deficiency: Classification of 105 Mutations and a General System for Genotype-Based Prediction of Metabolic Phenotype. Am J Hum Genet. 1998;63:71-79.

Guthrie R, Susi A. A simple Phenylalanine method for detecting Phenylketonuria in large populations of newborn infants. Pediatrics. 1963;32:338-343.

Güttler F, Guldberg KF. Mutations in the phenylalanine hydroxylase gene: genetic determinants for the phenotypic variability of hyperphenylalaninemia. Acta Paediatr. 1994;407 Suppl:46-56.

Halbesma N, Bakker SJ, Jansen DF et al. High protein intake associates with cardiovascular events but not with loss of renal function. J Am Soc Nephrol. 2009;20:1797-1804.

Hartwig C, Gal A, Santer R, Ullrich K, Finckh U, Kreienkamp H-J. Elevated phenylalanine levels interfere with neurite outgrowth stimulated by the neuronal cell adhesion molecule L1 in vitro. FEBS Letters. 2006;580:3489-3492.

Hidalgo IJ, Borchardt RT. Transport of a large neutral amino acid (phenylalanine) in a human intestinal epithelial cell line: Caco-2. Biochim Biophys Acta. 1990;1028:25-30.

Hoeks MP, den Heijer M, Janssen MC. Adult issues in phenylketonuria. Neth J Med. 2009;67:2-7.

Hughes JV, Johnson TC. Experimentally induced and natural recovery from the effects of phenylalanine on brain protein synthesis. Biochim Biophys Acta. 1978;517:473-485.

Kambham N, Markowitz GS, Valeri AM. Obesity-related glomerulopathy: an emerging epidemic. Kidney Int. 2001;59:1498-1509.

King AJ, Levey AS. Dietary protein and renal function. J Am Soc Nephrol. 1993;3:1723-1737.

Kure S, Hou DC, Ohura T, et al. Tetrahydrobiopterin-responsive phenylalanine hydroxylase deficiency. J Pediatr. 1999;135:375-378.

Kure S, Sato K, Fujii K, et al. Wild-type phenylalanine hydroxylase activity is enhanced by tetrahydrobiopterin supplementation in vivo: an implication for therapeutic basis of tetrahydrobiopterin-responsive phenylalanine hydroxylase deficiency. Mol Genet Metab. 2004;83:150-156.

Leandro J, Leandro P, Flatmark T. Heterotetrameric forms of human phenylalanine hydroxylase: co-expression of wild-type and mutant forms in a bicistronic system. Biochim Biophys Acta. 2011;1812:602-612.

Lee P, Treacy EP, Crombez E, et al. Safety and efficacy of 22 weeks of treatment with sapropterin dihydrochloride in patients with phenylketonuria. Am J Med Genet. 2008;146A:2851-2859.

Levy HL, Milanowski A, Chakrapani A, et al. Efficacy of sapropterin dihydrochloride (tetrahydrobiopterin, 6R-BH4) for reduction of phenylalanine concentration in patients with phenylketonuria: a phase III randomised placebo-controlled study. Lancet. 2007;370:504-510.

Lichter-Konecki U, Hipke CM, Konecki DS. Human phenylalanine hydroxylase gene expression in kidney and other nonhepatic tissues. Mol Genet Metab. 1999;67:308-316.

Lim K, van Calcar SC, Nelson KL, Gleason ST, Ney DM. Acceptable low-phenylalanine foods and beverages can be made with glycomacropeptide from cheese whey for individuals with PKU. Mol Genet Metab. 2007;92:176-178.

MacDonald A, Gokmen-Ozel H, van Rijn M, Burgard P. The reality of dietary compliance in the management of phenylketonuria. J Inherit Metab Dis. 2010;33:665-670.

MacDonald A, Rocha JC, van Rijn M, Feillet F. Nutrition in phenylketonuria. Mol Genet Metab. 2011;104 Suppl:S10-S18.

Machill G, Grimm U, Ahlbehrendt I, Bührdel P, Tittelbach-Helmrich W, Naumann A, Böhme HJ, Seidlitz G, Schneider T. Results of selective screening for inborn errors of metabolism in the former East Germany. Eur J Pediatr. 1994;153 Suppl 1:S14-S16.

MacLeod EL, Clayton MK, van Calcar SC, Ney DM. Breakfast with glycomacropeptide compared with amino acids suppresses plasma ghrelin levels in individuals with phenylketonuria. Mol Genet Metab. 2010;100:303-308.

Matalon R, Michals-Matalon K, Bhatia G, et al. Double blind placebo control trial of large neutral amino acids in treatment of PKU: effect on blood phenylalanine. J Inherit Metab Dis. 2007;30:153-158.

Mathias D, Bickel H. Follow-up study of 16 years neonatal screening for inborn errors of metabolism in West Germany. Eur J Pediatr. 1986;145:310-312.

McKean CM. The effects of high phenylalanine concentrations on serotonin and catecholamine metabolism in the human brain. Brain Res. 1972;47:469-476.

McNeill E, Keith M. Channon KM. The role of tetrahydrobiopterin in inflammation and cardiovascular disease. Thromb Haemost. 2012;108:832-839.

Mönch E, Herrmann ME, Brösicke H, Schöffer A, Keller M. Utilisation of amino acid mixtures in adolescents with phenylketonuria. Eur J Pediatr. 1996;155 Suppl 1:S115-S120.

Mönch E, Link R. Diagnostik und Therapie bei angeborenen Stoffwechselstörungen. SPS Verlagsgesellschaft, 2006, 2. Auflage.

Moyle JJ, Fox AM, Arthur M, Bynevelt M, Burnett JR. Meta-analysis of neuropsychological symptoms of adolescents and adults with PKU. Neuropsychol Rev. 2007;17:91-101.

Muntau AC, Gersting SW. Phenylketonuria as a model for protein misfolding diseases and for the development of next generation orphan drugs for patients with inborn errors of metabolism. J Inherit Metab Dis. 2010;33:649-658.

Muntau AC, Röschinger W, Habich M, et al. Tetrahydrobiopterin as an alternative treatment for mild phenylketonuria. N Engl J Med. 2002;347:2122-2132.

Nielsen JB, Nielsen KE, Güttler F. Tetrahydrobiopterin responsiveness after extended loading test of 12 Danish PKU patients with the Y414C mutation. J Inherit Metab Dis. 2010;33:9-16.

Pérez-Dueñas B, Valls-Solé J, Fernández-Alvarez E, et al. Characterization of tremor in phenylketonuric patients. J Neurol. 2005;252:1328-1334.

Pietz J, Kreis R, Rupp A, et al. Large neutral amino acids block phenylalanine transport into brain tissue in patients with phenylketonuria. J Clin Invest. 1999;103:1169-1178.

Pitt D. The natural history of untreated phenylketonuria. Med J Aust. 1971;1:378-383.

Ponzone A, Guardamagna O, Dianzani I, et al. Catalytic activity of tetrahydrobiopterin in dihydropteridine reductase deficiency and indications for treatment. Pediatr Res. 1993;33:125-128.

Porkert M, Sher S, Reddy U, et al. Tetrahydrobiopterin: a novel antihypertensive therapy. J Hum Hypertens. 2008;22:401-407.

Ribas GS, Sitta A, Wajner M, Vargas CR. Oxidative stress in phenylketonuria: what is the evidence? Cell Mol Neurobiol. 2011;31:653-662.

Sarkissian CN, Gámez A, Wang L, et al. Preclinical evaluation of multiple species of PEGylated recombinant phenylalanine ammonia lyase for the treatment of phenylketonuria. Proc Natl Acad Sci USA. 2008;105:20894-20899.

Schindeler S, Ghosh-Jerath S, Thompson S, et al. The effects of large neutral amino acid supplements in PKU: an MRS and neuropsychological study. Mol Genet Metab. 2007;91:48-54.

Schumacher U, Lukacs Z, Kaltschmidt C, et al. High concentrations of phenylalanine stimulate peroxisome proliferator-activated receptor gamma: implications for the pathophysiology of phenylketonuria. Neurobiol Dis. 2008;32:385-390.

Schwahn B, Mokov E, Scheidhauer K, Lettgen B, Schönau E. Decreased trabecular bone mineral density in patients with phenylketonuria measured by peripheral quantitative computed tomography. Acta Paediatr. 1998;7:61-63.

Scriver CR, Kaufman S. Phenylalanine hydroxylase deficiency in: Scriver CR, Beaudet AL, Sly W, Valle D, Childs B, Vogelstein B (Eds.). The Metabolic and Molecular Basis of Inherited Disease, 2001. McGraw-Hill New York, pp. 1667-1724.

Singh RH, Quirk ME, Douglas TD, Brauchla MC. BH(4) therapy impacts the nutrition status and intake in children with phenylketonuria: 2-year follow-up. J Inherit Metab Dis. 2010;33:689-695.

Solverson P, Murali SG, Brinkman AS, et al. Glycomacropeptide, a low-phenylalanine protein isolated from cheese whey, supports growth and attenuates metabolic stress in the murine model of phenylketonuria. Am J Physiol Endocrinol Metab. 2012;302:E885-895.

Staudigl M, Gersting SW, Danecka MK, et al. The interplay between genotype, metabolic state and cofactor treatment governs phenylalanine hydroxylase function and drug response. Hum Mol Genet. 2011;20:2628-2641.

Stéphenne X, Debray FG, Smets F, et al. Hepatocyte transplantation using the domino concept in a child with Tetrabiopterin non-responsive phenylketonuria. Cell Transplant. 2012;21:2765-2770.

Thöny B. Long-term correction of murine phenylketonuria by viral gene transfer: liver versus muscle. J Inherit Metab Dis. 2010;DOI: 10.1007/s10545-010-9044-3.

Trefz FK, Scheible D, Frauendienst-Egger G. Long-term follow-up of patients with phenylketonuria receiving tetrahydrobiopterin treatment. J Inherit Metab Dis. 2010;DOI: 10.1007/s10545-010-9058-x.

van Calcar SC, MacLeod EL, Gleason ST, et al. Improved nutritional management of phenylketonuria by using a diet containing glycomacropeptide compared with amino acids. Am J Clin Nutr. 2009;89:1068-1077

Waisbren SE, Noel K, Fahrbach K, et al. Phenylalanine blood levels and clinical outcomes in phenylketonuria: a systematic literature review and meta-analysis. Mol Genet Metab. 2007;92:63-70.

Walter JH, Lee PJ, Burgard P. Hyperphenylalaninaemia in: Fernandes J, Saudubray JM, van den Berghe G, Walter JH (Eds.). Inborn Metabolic Diseases: Diagnosis and Treatment. 2006. Springer Verlag Heidelberg, pp:221-231.

Walter JH, White FJ, Hall SK, et al. How practical are recommendations for dietary control in phenylketonuria? Lancet. 2002;360:55-57.

Weglage J, Ullrich K, Pietsch M, Fünders B, Zass R, Koch HG. Untreated non-phenylketonuric-hyperphenylalaninaemia: intellectual and neurological outcome. Eur J Pediatr. 1996;155 Suppl 1:S26-28.

Weigel C, Rauh M, Kiener C, Rascher W, Knerr I. Effects of various dietary amino acid preparations for phenylketonuric patients on the metabolic profiles along with postprandial insulin and ghrelin responses. Ann Nutr Metab. 2007;51:352-358.

White JE, Kronmal RA, Acosta PB. Excess weight among children with phenylketonuria. J Am Coll Nutr. 1982;1:293-303.

Zager RA, Johannes G, Tuttle SE, Sharma HM. Acute amino acid nephrotoxicity. J Lab Clin Med. 1983;101:130–140

Zhao YY, Liu J, Cheng XL, Bai X, Lin RC. Urinary metabonomics study on biochemical changes in an experimental model of chronic renal failure by adenine based on UPLC Q-TOF/MS. Clin Chim Acta. 2012;413:642-649.

Ziesch B, Weigel J, Thiele A, et al. Tetrahydrobiopterin (BH4) in PKU: effect on dietary treatment, metabolic control, and quality of life. J Inherit Metab Dis. 2012;35:983-992.

Zschocke J, Mallory JP, Eiken HG, Nevin NC. Phenylketonuria and the peoples of Northern Ireland. Hum Genet. 1997;100:189-194.

Zurflüh MR, Fiori L, Fiege B, et al. Pharmacokinetics of orally administered tetrahydrobiopterin in patients with phenylalanine hydroxylase deficiency. J Inherit Metab Dis. 2006;29:725-731.

Danksagung

Mein herzlichster Dank gilt allen, die mich während meiner klinischen Arbeit und meiner Forschungsarbeit und damit auf dem Weg zu meiner Habilitation begleitet und unterstützt haben. Allen voran danke ich Herrn Dr. Jürgen Herwig, Herrn Dr. Adrian Sewell und Herrn Prof. Dr. Hansjosef Böhles aus der Universitätskinderklinik in Frankfurt, die mir als Erste den Stoffwechsel nahe gebracht haben und denen es gelang, meine Begeisterung für dieses Gebiet zu entfachen.

Aus der Kinderklinik der Charité Berlin danke ich Herrn Prof. Dr. Eberhard Mönch für die jahrelange enge Zusammenarbeit und die gemeinsame Betreuung vieler Patienten mit Phenylketonurie und anderen angeborenen Stoffwechselerkrankungen. Herrn Prof. Dr. Gerhard Gaedicke danke ich für sein großes Vertrauen, das er stets in mich und in meine Arbeit gesetzt hat.

Ich danke meinen beiden Doktorandinnen Sylvia Roloff und Jeanne-Marie Berger für ihre unermüdliche und sehr engagierte Arbeit sowohl in der Durchführung ihrer Promotionsarbeiten als auch in der Datenerhebung für die verschiedenen BH4-Studien.

Frau Dr. Barbara Vetter danke ich für ihre Unterstützung bei den molekulargenetischen Analysen der PKU-Patienten. Herrn Prof. Dr. Andreas E. Kulozik danke ich für die gemeinsame erfolgreiche Arbeit zu den PKU-Genotypen.

Herrn Prof. Dr. Uwe Querfeld danke ich für die sehr produktive und engagierte gemeinsame Arbeit zu den Nierenschädigungen bei Patienten mit PKU. Ebenso möchte ich Frau Dr. Jutta Gellermann für ihre Hilfe bei der Untersuchung der Nierenfunktion der PKU-Patienten danken.

Ich danke Herrn Prof. Dr. Nenad Blau aus dem Kinderspital in Zürich, jetzt Universitätskinderklinik Heidelberg, sehr herzlich für die gute Zusammenarbeit.

Herrn Prof. Dr. Johan van Hove der University of Colorado in Aurora/USA danke ich für die sehr inspirierende Kooperation bei den Untersuchungen zur Glyzin-Enzephalopathie.

Ich danke allen Kolleginnen und Kollegen aus unserem Stoffwechsel-Team, vor allem Frau Christine Gebauer, die unzählige Diätprotokolle unserer PKU Patienten berechnet hat.

Allen PKU-Patienten und deren Familien danke ich für die Teilnahme an den verschiedenen Studien und Untersuchungen.

Schlussendlich und von ganzem Herzen danke ich meiner Familie und all meinen Freunden für ihr unendliches Verständnis, ihre dauerhafte Unterstützung und ihre nie endenden Ermutigungen.

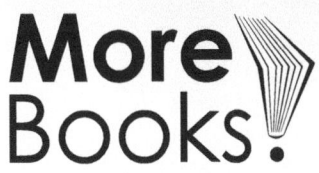
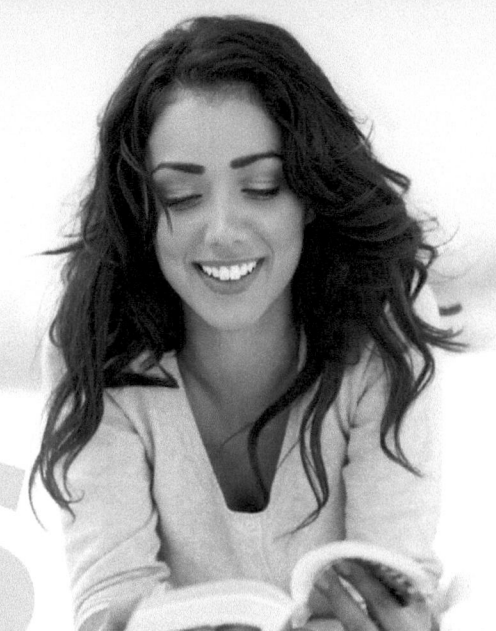

i want morebooks!

Buy your books fast and straightforward online - at one of world's fastest growing online book stores! Environmentally sound due to Print-on-Demand technologies.

Buy your books online at
www.get-morebooks.com

Kaufen Sie Ihre Bücher schnell und unkompliziert online – auf einer der am schnellsten wachsenden Buchhandelsplattformen weltweit! Dank Print-On-Demand umwelt- und ressourcenschonend produziert.

Bücher schneller online kaufen
www.morebooks.de

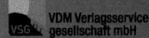 VDM Verlagsservicegesellschaft mbH
Heinrich-Böcking-Str. 6-8   Telefon: +49 681 3720 174   info@vdm-vsg.de
D - 66121 Saarbrücken   Telefax: +49 681 3720 1749 www.vdm-vsg.de

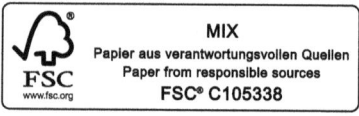

Printed by Books on Demand GmbH, Norderstedt / Germany